HOT FLASHES AND HALF IRONMANS

MIDDLE-AGED ENDURANCE ATHLETICS MEETS THE HORMONALLY CHALLENGED

PF HUTCHINS

SKIPJACK PUBLISHING

FREE EBOOKS

Before you begin reading, you can snag a free Pamela Fagan Hutchins ebook starter library by joining her mailing list at https://pamelafaganhutchins.com/sign-up-for-pamela-fagan-hutchins-author-newsletter/.

I DON'T ASK MUCH.

{Before you start, you can snag an exclusive, free Pamela Fagan Hutchins' *What Doesn't Kill You* mystery novella by joining her mailing list at http://eepurl.com/lq-bP, if you wanna.}

They say youth is wasted on the young. They are full of it. Youth is too full of angst and drama for me. Give me middle age, wisdom, and a healthy libido any day. Give me some crappy life experiences so I'll recognize awesome when it lands in my lap. Give me cellulite and wrinkles so I can get the hell over myself. Give me boredom so I can appreciate a challenge, and give me a failed marriage to humble me. Give me hot flashes and migraines so I can enjoy feeling good the rest of the time.

And then, then . . . give me a hot day in June. Let me fill our beater Suburban to its capacity with tweens and teens, some of them mine, some of them his. Let us pick up my second and last husband at the airport after a long and tiring business trip, let us giggle all the way home and nearly burst with the pressure of our shared secret. We have a surprise for him, you see.

We whisk him home to his bicycle and tri bag.

"What's this?" he asks, dark circles under his camouflage-colored eyes. Eyes that are sparkling now between the red lines.

"Here!" his daughter Liz cries, unable to hold it in any longer. She waggles her hand at Clark and Susanne, who pull t-shirts on over their heads. The hand-ironed custom logo is slightly askew on each of them. It reads "The Eric Ralph Hutchins First Annual Invitational Triathlon" above a (really bad) picture of Eric.

"Those are great, guys, thanks," he says as Liz hands him his and he slips it on.

But that's not all. "Put your swimsuit on, honey, because the race starts in fifteen minutes," I say.

Now he's grinning ear to ear. We all jump on our bikes and pedal over to the Marilyn Estates pool. We swim ten thrashing, splashing, laughing laps of the tiny rectangle of water. We race our motley crew of bicycles around the block. And we finish by running figure eights around the trees in the park by the pool. Fifteen minutes later, we each get a trophy, with awards for first (Liz), second (Eric), poutiest (Susanne), goofiest (Clark), and best-looking, AKA last (me). We've attracted quite a crowd, and they cheer as the kids present the awards.

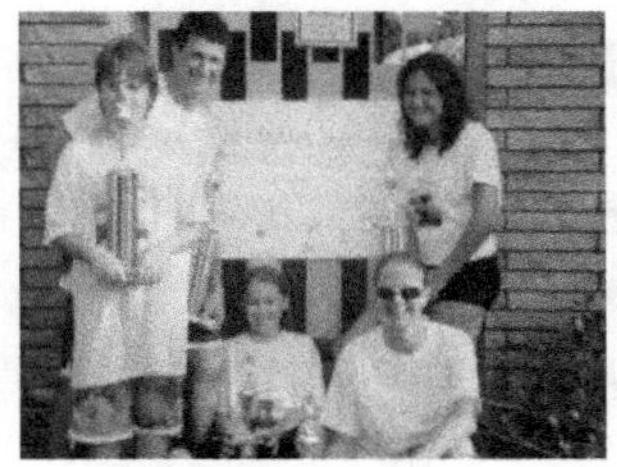

My husband doesn't seem tired anymore. He looks like the luckiest middle-aged man in the history of the world. Although he doesn't look middle-aged, which makes me the luckiest middle-aged woman ever.

This. Give me this. Or something a whole lot like it. Give me beautiful days together, active and alive, happy and feeling fifteen instead of closing in on fifty.

This, or something like it.

PUTTING THE FUN INTO DYSFUNCTIONAL

I am a planner. I plan and schedule and plot, much to the delight of my engineer/triathlete husband, who loves to live by a plan. Even more, he loves for me to make the plan and then for us both to live by it. And what he loves most of all is when the plan I make and we live by includes a healthy dose of us bicycling and swimming together. I believe a plan is a structure to make reasonable changes in, while Eric casts his plans in cement. Obviously, I am right, so there usually isn't much of a problem.

But I did not plan what happened to us in the Good Old Summertime Classic, a sixty-nine-mile bicycle ride along some of our most favorite cycling roads anywhere. The bike route runs in and around Fayetteville, Texas, and includes the tiny old town of Roundtop. We had trained for it. We had talked about it with joy and reverence. Eric even accidentally went to get our packets a full week before they were available for pickup. (Don't ask.)

The night before the race, I developed a PMS {Technically, I suffer from premenstrual dysphoric disorder, but try to say "I'm feeling PMDDy" or "I'm really PMDDing right now." Yeah. It doesn't exactly roll off the tongue. PMDD is a severe and sometimes disabling form of PMS.} hormonal migraine. Because it was the middle of the night, I took one of my gentler migraine prescriptions, hoping that this pill plus sleep would be all I needed. But when I woke up at 5:00 a.m. to the mother of all migraines, I caved in and went for the elephant tranquilizer. When morning came, I was so nauseous that I couldn't eat. My husband, a man of immense patience and even greater kindness, suggested we stay home. But we had made a plan, so I got in the car. I theorized that I had no idea now how I would feel in two and a half hours—but I kinda did know, and just didn't want to admit it.

I should have listened to my husband.

On the way to the race, driving in the dark, the unthinkable happened. I had my head on Eric's shoulder, sweetly sleeping (make that "snoring and drooling under the influence of the elephant pill"), when he let out a tiny swear word. Actually, I believe it started with an F, and was preceded by the word "mother," and that his voice blasted through my cranium and echoed madly inside my impaired brain.

"What happened?" I screamed, heart pounding, hand clutching throat, eyes sweeping the road for signs of the apocalypse.

"I hit a cardinal."

OH MY GOD. HE HIT A CARDINAL.

Since the time he could speak, my husband has proclaimed himself a fan of the ~~ChicagoPhoenixSt. Louis~~ Arizona Cardinals football team. His screen saver at work has always been a giant Cardinal ~~head~~ logo, until very recently when he finally switched it to a picture of us, under teensy-tinsy little applications of subtle pressure from me. He watched their 2009 playoff game at 2:00 a.m. from his hotel room in Libya through a webcam picture of our TV on his laptop. He collects cardinals and Cardinal paraphernalia and insists on displaying them prominently in our bedroom, which is painted Cardinal red.

Despite his lifelong obsession, Eric had never seen an actual live cardinal bird until we moved to Houston. Growing up in the U.S. Virgin Islands, he'd caught glimpses of them on TV, and he pictured them as red, fierce . . . and large.

One day while unpacking boxes in our new house, I saw a male cardinal through the window. Nonchalantly, I called out to my sweetie, "Hey, Eric, there's a cardinal in our bird feeder."

Eric, whose physique looks like you would expect it to after twenty years of triathlon and cycling, pounded into the living room like a rhino instead of his usual cheetah self, wearing an expectant grin and not much else.

"WHERE IS IT?"

Lost for words, I pointed out the front window and prayed the elderly woman next door was not walking past our house.

"It's awfully small." (That was Eric that said that, not the elderly neighbor.)

He was crestfallen. The mighty cardinal was a tiny slip of a bird.

Back to the car: ear-splitting expletives and wife under the influence.   "Honey, I didn't feel an impact. Are you sure you didn't miss it?" I asked.

"They're awfully small birds," he said.

Ahhhh, good point. We drove on, somberly. We arrived at the race. I stumbled off to the bathroom. When I came back, Eric was crouched in front of the grill of our car. I joined him, confused. He held up a handful of tiny red feathers.

I swear it was the drugs, but I burst out laughing. "You, you of all people, you killed a *cardinal*?"

He glared at me as he picked out the brightest of the small feathers and tucked it reverently into the chest strap of his heart monitor. "I'm going to carry this feather with me in tribute, the whole way."

So we got on our bikes: me, wobbly, cotton-mouthed, and somewhat delirious; Eric, solemn and determined. This, the ride for the cardinal, would be the ride of his life. Sixty-nine miles to the glory of the cardinal.

I made it all of about two miles before I apologized. "I'm anaerobic, and we're only going twelve miles per hour on a flat. My neck and back are seizing up. I don't know if it's drugs or hormones, but I'm really whack."

"You can do it, honey. We came all this way. Now we're riding for a higher purpose."

I gave it my best, I really did, but a few miles later after a succession of hills where going up with a racing heartbeat was only slightly less awful than cruising down with a seriously messed-up sense of balance, I pulled to a stop. "I've never quit before, but I can't do it today, love."

A beautiful male cardinal swooped across the road in front of us. Eric bit his lip. "I understand. Do you want to flag a SAG [support and aid] wagon?"

"I can make it back if we just take it easy. I'm sorry, honey."

My husband treated me like a princess that day, but all the excitement had drained out of him. This race was not to be, and a teacup-sized bird had sacrificed his life in vain because I'd overdosed on Immitrex and ruined the plan. The waste of it all, the waste of a day, the waste of a life—it was hard to overcome. But Eric tried; I'll give him credit for that, the man really tried.

That night, after we did a make-up ride on the trainers while we watched *We Are Marshall* (interrupted occasionally by Eric's sobs, because the only thing worse than a dead cardinal is a dead football player), I pulled our sheets out of the drier and brought them into our room. Eric, wearing his new Fayetteville Good Old Summertime T-shirt, helped me put the warm, clean cotton on the bed.

As we hoisted the sheets in the air to spread them out over the mattress, a tiny red feather shot straight up toward the light and wafted down slowly, back and forth, back and forth, until, pushed by the soft breeze of our ceiling fan, it landed on the pillow on Eric's side of the bed.

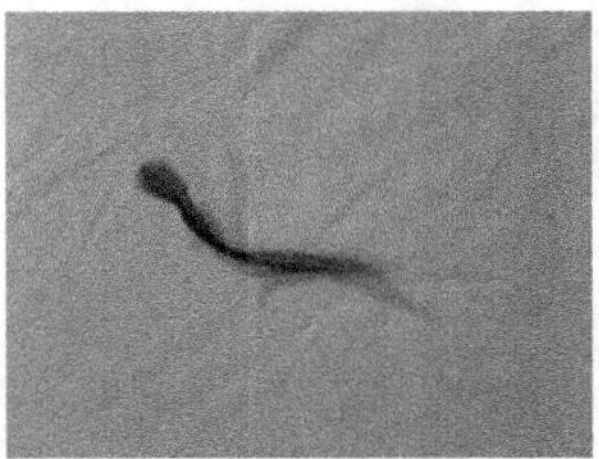

Above: Actual cardinal feather on Eric's pillow.

Steeling myself for the worst, I shot a glance at him to see if he had noticed. I did not exhale. Maybe I had time to brush it off quickly? Too late—he was staring at the feather. "Is that damn bird going to haunt me for the rest of my life now?" he asked. But he smiled.

Now I could breathe. And tease. "Probably. You did senselessly murder a cardinal, Eric."

And he laughed.

WEREWOLF OF HOUSTON

As a nearing-middle-age woman whose athletic second husband wanted her to triathlon with him, I seemed well-enough equipped. I had run cross-country as a teen and continued in adulthood. I'd come close to doing the New York Marathon in 2001 before succumbing to an ill-timed bout of salmonella. I'd even dabbled in sprint triathlons a few times. My will was iron and my health superb.

Until I hit the age of forty. Boom, boom, out went the lights. My PMS or PMDD or whatever it was went from laughingly bad to frighteningly worse. I began a monthly descent into a hell I shared with my husband that included week-long migraines, night sweats, complete irrationality, unexplained anxiety, and, most troubling, episodes of violent rage followed by a fugue state of crushing guilt and unstoppable tears. I gained a quick fifteen pounds and kept piling it on, and my whole body hurt like I had fibromyalgia.

After it ended, I would reel for days in exhaustion. But when it was over, it was over, and I was normal, even serenely happy, until it hit again. While it was happening, though . . . whoa, Nellie . . . we didn't even know me, and no object in our bedroom was safe from my intent to throw or slam it down. I lost my voice from screaming more often than I want to remember.

It took us about four months to realize that this was not an aberration, and that it was sometimes happening more than once a cycle. Yet, as moody as I was, I was not depressed; I've been depressed, and this was rage, not sadness.

It sucked. And not only did I feel awful, but I didn't even want to get out of bed, much less get on a bike or into the water. I put my running shoes in the back of the closet for a week or more each month.

One month when it hit, I packed a suitcase.

"Where the heck do you think you're going?" Eric asked.

Cue the irrationality. "I need to get away from me. Away from how I feel," I answered.

Luckily, Eric was able to talk me out of this great plan. What else to do, though, but hide? I had no idea what was wrong or how to stop it, if it even could be stopped. I wanted to go to sleep for a very long time. Until it was over. And if that didn't work, death sounded good. For a few days each month, it sounded very, very good.

I spent months reading, researching, consulting physicians, and experimenting as I tried to attack the problem from every conceivable angle. Meanwhile, we sheltered our kids from the impact (think *Pamela in a padded room*). But I couldn't save Eric from it. He tried to do everything for me, sometimes from a continent away, and often missed precious hours at the job we both needed for him to do so well at, as he worried that something really awful would happen during my bad days. There were times I couldn't handle simple human interactions, whether it be with strangers, family, or friends. There were days I couldn't do my day job over "nothing but hormones"—me, a woman who prides herself on doing whatever is needed, pulling all-nighters, muscling through anything; a woman who absolutely knows how critical her income is to her family. I hid in my room and isolated the world from the poison of me.

I don't know if it would have made it better to be in on the joke. Apparently, it is not enough that women pay for the apple incident through childbirth and lower equivalent hourly wages. No, we must also pay through a rite of passage *so misunderstood* that many doctors (and definitely mine) poo-poo its very existence: perimenopause.

Most women know to expect menopause, or the cessation of menses, at around the age of fifty. But when you turned thirty-five, did *your* gynecologist start discussing with you the dramatic changes you might experience over the next fifteen or so years? Did she help you prepare for them, and warn you against thinking you had lost your flippin' mind? None of mine did, and I'd had several since my mid thirties.

Here's how the Mayo Clinic defines perimenopause on its website:

"Perimenopause, also called the menopausal transition, is the interval in which a woman's body makes a natural shift from more-or-less regular cycles of ovulation and menstruation toward permanent infertility, or menopause.

"Women start perimenopause at different ages. In your 40s, or even as early as your 30s, you may start noticing the signs. Your periods may become irregular—longer, shorter, heavier or lighter, sometimes more and sometimes less than 28 days apart. You may also experience menopause-like symptoms, such as hot flashes, sleep problems and vaginal dryness. Treatments are available to help ease these symptoms.

"Once you've gone through 12 consecutive months without a menstrual period, you've officially reached menopause, and the perimenopause period is over." {http://www.mayoclinic.com/health/peri menopause/DS00554}

The lucky perimenopausal women out there will experience a variety of symptoms that are mild to moderate, including these {Paraphrased, but originally researched at http://www.mayoclinic.com/health/perimenopause/DS00554}:

Menstrual irregularity. Ovulation and periods go haywire during perimenopause. Cycles become shorter or longer, closer together or farther apart, lighter or heavier, or, as with me, vary in all categories. If your menstrual cycle length changes by more than seven days, you are probably experiencing early perimenopause. If you miss two or more periods and have longer than 60 days between periods, you are probably in late perimenopause.

Hot flashes and sleep problems. The great majority of women will have hot flashes, usually during late perimenopause, although I had them early on. Hot flashes and night sweats can cause sleep problems, although women may have sleep problems during perimenopause anyway. The intensity, duration, and frequency of hot flashes and night sweats vary. I could fill a wading pool with a night sweat, but hot flashes for me weren't nearly as bad.

Mood changes. Ah, the famous "mood changes" of perimenopause: mood swings, irritability, or depression. Some experts think the sleep disruptions are the cause, and they caution that other factors besides the hormonal changes of perimenopause can cause mood changes. Yes, all probably true. And yet the hormonal changes of perimenopause can be the factor causing them as well. This, for me, was the worst symptom of all.

Vaginal and bladder problems. Make it stop! Your estrogen levels drop during perimenopause, and all kinds of yucky things may happen as a result, like loss of lubrication in vaginal tissues, which can make intercourse painful; vulnerability to urinary tract infections; and urinary incontinence. (Raising my hand for all three.)

Decreasing fertility. Ladies, beware. You can still get pregnant as long as you are having periods. However, fertility decreases during perimenopause.

Changes in sexual function. The good news here is that if you enjoyed sex before, you'll probably continue to enjoy it in perimenopause and beyond, although there is a chance that some women may experience a decrease in arousal level and sexual desire. This is about the only symptom category in which I am in the "lucky" group; no problems here.

Loss of bone. Take your calcium and vitamin D! Bone loss begins to occur faster than you can replace it during perimenopause. This puts you at a higher risk of osteoporosis. Every year my blood work shows a need for higher levels of calcium and vitamin D. I currently take 10,000 mg of D daily with 600 mg of calcium citrate, in addition to my multivitamin.

Changing cholesterol levels. It's not uncommon for women in perimenopause to discover unfavorable changes in blood cholesterol levels, including an increase in the "bad" cholesterol, low-density lipoprotein (LDL) cholesterol. This can contribute to an increased risk of heart disease, and the medical community believes it is tied to decreasing estrogen levels. The timing of the LDL increase is bad, as high-density lipoprotein (HDL) cholesterol—the "good" cholesterol—decreases in many women as they age, another factor contributing to possible heart disease. And, yes, my LDL went up and HDL went down at age 40.

Basically, perimenopause is like PMS on acid. The symptoms sneak up on you and are unpleasant and surprising, but somewhat controllable. Unfortunately, it's not as easy to self-diagnose as, say, a bleeding stump or a smallpox lesion. If no one prepares you to expect it, how do you even know it's OK to raise your hand and ask for help?

Most women can get some relief through a good diet, exercise, sunshine, sleep, stress reduction, and anger management. It helps to stay hydrated and to cut down on alcohol and caffeine. Supplements specifically designed for PMS, depression, or perimenopause can make a difference, and in more severe cases, some doctors prescribe low-dose birth control to even out the hormones (more on *that* later).

For some of us, though, the symptoms slip us into a terrifyingly altered mood. Irritation to the power of infinity. I'm pretty sure the first documented werewolf was one of my perimenopausal ancestors.

Would it have made it better if I had known this could happen? Yes. I was convinced that I was going insane, which was scary. I thought I was turning into Lizzie Borden, and I made Eric get rid of our ax. I started writing angry poetry {http://pamelahutchins.com/2011/01/25/gouge-your-eyes-out-poetry-slam/} If I'd have known, I could have sought the right solutions sooner. I certainly knew to start getting mammograms at age forty and to get annual pap smears; is it such a stretch to expect my gynecologists to gently question and educate me on the symptoms of hormonal changes and imbalance that, while not abnormal, did not have to affect me so greatly? I'm an extreme example with my werewolf-like symptoms, but I know now that many, many women endure these symptoms simply because no one has ever told them that they don't have to. No one has told them that *they aren't crazy and they aren't alone.*

I felt worse than I ever had in my life. My biggest fear though, was that I might be feeling the best I ever would again, that I was in a state of decline that was irreversible and far from rock bottom. And this was when I realized that, no matter what, I had to find a way to keep my inner athlete alive. Or bring her back to life, rather. She had taken her last breath months ago and was in dire need of mouth-to-mouth resuscitation.

BRING IT.

I didn't have this perimenopause thing licked yet, but I soldiered on, looking for the right defense to mount against the monthly hormonal assault. I was secure in knowing that I am loved and accepted. I kept my stress as low as possible. I improved my diet and started taking sleep aids. I ran my own human trials on perimenopause, anxiety, PMS, and depression supplements; it seemed unlikely they'd make me any worse. And in the non-hormonal times, I just worked harder, to make up for the time the werewolf stole from me.

And I started training for a Half Ironman triathlon.

It had taken me a while (about two years) to realize that my brand spanking-new husband wasn't about to do another endurance triathlon if I didn't do it with him. Before we were together, Eric immersed himself in triathlon and slappin' da bass, and when we got married, I thought my job was to enable him to keep that up. But I'd missed the point: sports and music had been his escape as much as his passion. He wasn't going to either one if I didn't do it with him.

When I finally figured that out, it made perfect sense, and I knew exactly what to do. Eric and I are the proud authors of our very own Relationship Operating Agreement, a document that encompasses our shared values, our commitments to each other, and our vision of our marriage. It read, in part, as follows: *Our relationship's purpose is to create a loving, nurturing, safe environment that enables us to make a positive, joyful difference in each other's lives and encourage each other's spiritual, emotional, and physical needs and development.*

So when Eric said this: "How about we train for a Half Ironman together?," I said this: "Absolutely."

But I didn't know if I was up for it. "Do you think I can do it?" One of my two life goals was to complete a marathon (the other was to write a book—check!), but I'd been exercising less and less as my monthly cycles had gotten worse.

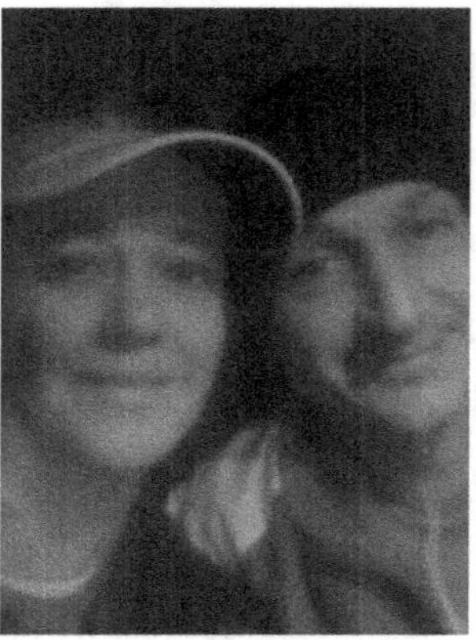

"I know you can. We'll start slow and build carefully."

My doubts receded fast. I am strange that way. "Bring it," I said. "Can we follow up with a marathon for me?"

Eric broke into his crooked smile. "I will trade you a Half Ironman for a marathon as many times as you want. You'll have to conquer a marathon to make a full Ironman, and that's what I really want us to do someday. Together."

Take it slow and *one step at a time* are not catchphrases at our house.

"Could we get the cool M-dot Ironman tattoos on our ankles?" I asked, skipping mentally over the months of grueling training and drilling to the really important issue of race bling.

"Yah, mon," he said. "It's practically required."

"Perfect," I replied.

THEY BROKE THE MOLD
WHEN THEY MADE ME.

As I contemplated training for a Half Ironman, I knew I'd need to contain the horrors of my hormones. I went to my general practitioner, who sent me to my gynecologist. I visited Dr. Gyno in her fancy schmancy high-rise clinic in the Medical Center area near Rice University and laid it out in brutal and humiliating detail, pleading for her help.

"Do you think it's perimenopause?" I asked.

"Well, you're just too young for menopause symptoms. We should put you on antidepressants," she said.

"But I'm not depressed. Why would I take something I don't need?" I asked.

This did not sit well with me. Was she offering me a placebo to placate me? I was having serious problems. I needed serious assistance.

"Well, maybe not antidepressants, then. I can put you on birth control to even out your hormones. This helps some women."

"My husband has had a vasectomy. I don't really need birth control. Is this what you would do if you were me, though?" I asked her.

"Yes," she said.

"All right, then. I'm willing to try anything."

This was the sum of her contribution to solving my health crisis.

Nothing about diet, sleep, exercise, or supplements. As I reflected on everything I had read about perimenopause, I wondered how she could discount my story and my symptoms. Apparently, I didn't fit the cookie-cutter parameters that her experience and education had primed her to expect. But she had the ability to prescribe medication, and I needed to try something. The many supplements I had tried did not seem to make a dent. So I tried her low-dose birth control strategy.

And everything that had already gone from bad to worse went *nuclear*, all month long. I couldn't take it. I stopped after the first cycle and counted myself lucky that I hadn't hurt myself or anyone else during those twenty-eight days.

I had no idea what to do next.

I LOVE ME A PLAN.

Come hell or high hormones, Eric and I were going to do a Half Ironman. And because anything worth doing is better done with a plan, we made one.

We based our training on Trifuel's 70.3 training plan, which was developed by Matt Lieto, a professional triathlete and coach {http://www.mattlieto.com/}. The plan spanned twenty weeks and included three swims, three runs, and three bikes for six days of every week, with one day of rest. It assumed that we were starting as intermediate triathletes with a good base of fitness, and it ramped up fast, requiring twelve to fifteen hours a week, which meant nearly an hour of extra sleep each night for us.

For all you non-triathletes, a little tri info might be in order. Triathlons come in several models, but all include a swim, a bicycle, and a run segment, in that order. The swim zaps your energy and the bicycle burns out your quads. By the time you run, your legs feel like bricks; hence, running after biking is often called a brick.

The shortest triathlons are sprints. The swim distance in a sprint is usually about 800 meters, the bicycle approximately 12 miles, and the run 3 miles. Intermediate triathlons are Olympic distance, with a 1500-meter swim, 24-mile bike, and 6-mile run. I was training for a Half Ironman, known also as a 70.3, which is named for its distance in miles: 1.2-mile swim, 56-mile bike, and 13.1-mile run. It is exactly half the distance of a full Ironman, also known as a 140.6: 2.4-mile swim, 112-mile bike, and a full 26.2-mile marathon tagged on the end just for fun. .

We found the perfect event: the second annual Longhorn Half Ironman outside Austin, Texas. It was twenty-three weeks away, which gave us three weeks to focus on our (my) base fitness before we started the twenty-week stretch.

But after months of hormone poisoning, I couldn't keep up with Eric. I had spent way too much time feeding my hormones buttery popcorn while feeling sorry for myself. Still, I knew that underneath my recently fluffy middle and thighs was a strong woman. I was an experienced runner and a natural bicyclist.

My hurdle was the swim. I had grave doubts about my ability to do it without drowning, much less within the time limit. My upper-body strength was poor. The impact of my crazy hormones reduced the range of motion in my neck. The migraines nauseated me, which made freestyle breathing a nightmare. And I hated, hated, hated being wet and cold. I don't know who dreaded our early swims more, me or Eric, due to my ugly mood swings. But he (somewhat) patiently coached me. It was a huge boon to have a live-in coach, and to be part of our own two-person tri team.

If he could handle me, I could handle the swim. I dug deeper to find the strength I needed.

THERE'S NOTHING UNDER
THE CANOE, HONEY.

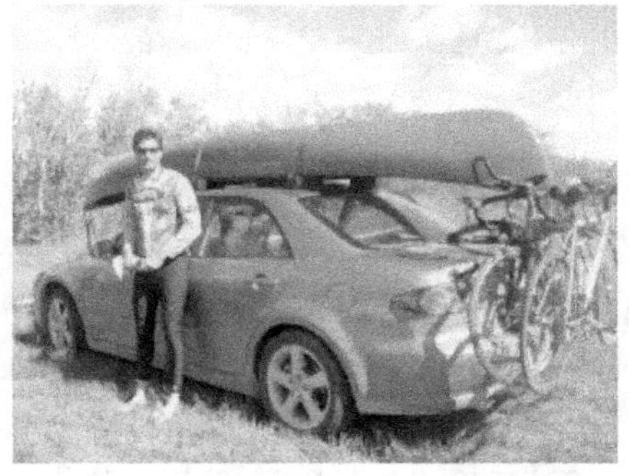

Above: This is how we roll.

Eric and I had scheduled our long-postponed honeymoon for Montana in June, which, we were surprised to discover, still felt like the dead of winter. (We hail from the Caribbean and Houston, Texas.) Since doing the swim portion of our training would not be possible during our two weeks of love in the Great White North, we needed to find an upper-body strength and aerobic substitute. Without taking the weather into account, we decided that canoeing or kayaking would suffice.

So off we traipsed to an adorable bed-and-breakfast near Yellowstone, chosen because the owner advertised healthy, organic food.

The beets, quinoa, and cauliflower kugel we were served for breakfast weren't exactly what we'd hoped for, but we felt fantastic, and we were fueled up for the honeymoon and the Half Ironman training alike.

Our "Surprise! We're vegetarian!" B&B sat near a tundra lake. For those of you who have not seen a tundra lake, imagine a beautiful lake in a mountain clearing surrounded by tall evergreens. Picture deer drinking from its crystalline waters, and hear the ducks quacking greetings to each other as they cruise its glassy surface. Smell the pine needles in the air, fresh and earthy.

Well, it's nothing like that.

A tundra lake is in the highlands, no doubt, but the similarity stops there: no trees, no windbreak, no calm surface, and no scenery. Instead, it's an ice-chunk-filled, white-capped pit of black water extending straight down to hell, stuck smack dab in the middle of a rock-strewn wasteland. Other than that, it's terrific.

Maybe it was because we were newlyweds, but somehow Eric intuited that I would love nothing more than to canoe this lake in forty-degree weather and thirty-five-mph winds, wearing sixty-seven layers of movement-restricting, water-absorbent clothing. Maybe it was because we were newlyweds, but I somehow assumed that because he knew of my dark water phobia and hatred of the cold (anything below seventy degrees), I was in good hands. My new husband assured me this lake was perfect for tandem canoeing.

So we drove across the barren terrain to the lake. Eric was bouncy. I was unable to make my mouth form words other than "You expect me to get in that @#$%&&*$* canoe on that @#$%&&*$* lake?"

I promise, he is smarter than this will sound. And that I am just as bitchy as I will sound. In my family, we call my behavior being the bell cow, as in "She who wears the bell leads the herd—and takes no shit from other cows."

Eric answered, "Absolutely, honey. It'll be great. Here, help me get the canoe in the water. I'd take it off the car myself, but with that wind, whew, it's like a sail. Careful not to dump it over; it's reallllly cold in there. Not like that, love. Where are you going? Did I say something wrong?"

The only response I gave him was the slam of the car door. Anger gave way to the tears that pricked the corners of my eyes. I stewed in my thoughts. I knew I had to try to canoe. I couldn't quit before I started. We were training. If I didn't do it, Eric wouldn't do it, and that wasn't fair of me.

I got out of the car. Eric was dragging the canoe out of the water and trying to avoid looking like a red flag waving in front of me.

Super-rationally, I asked, "What are you doing?"

He said, "Well, I'm not going to make you do this."

"You're not making me. I'm scared. I hate this. I'll probably fall in and all you'll find is my frozen carcass next summer. But I'm going to do it."

My poor husband.

We paddled around the lake clockwise in the shallows where the waves were lowest, and I fought for breath. I'm not sure if it was the constriction of all the clothing layers or actual hyperventilation, but either way, I panted like a three-hundred-pound marathoner. It would have scared off any animal life within five miles, if you could have heard me over the wind. Suddenly, Eric shot me a wild-eyed look and started paddling furiously toward the center of the lake.

"You're going the wrong way!" I protested.

"I can't hear you," he shouted back.

"Turn around!"

"I can't turn around right now, I'm paddling."

"Eric Hutchins, turn the canoe back toward the shore!"

And as quickly as his mad dash for the deep had started, it stopped. He angled the canoe for the shoreline.

"What in the hell was that all about?" I asked.

"Nothing, love. I just needed to get my heart rate up."

I sensed the lie, but I couldn't prove it. My own heart raced as if I had been the one sprint-paddling. For once, though, I kept my mouth shut.

The waves grew higher. We paddled and paddled for what felt like hours, but made little forward progress against the wicked-cold wind.

"Eric, I really want out of the canoe."

"We're halfway. Hang in there."

"No. I want out right now. I'm scared. We're going to tip over. I can't breathe."

"How about we cut across the middle of lake and shave off some distance? That will get you to the shore faster."

"I WANT TO GO THE NEAREST SHORE RIGHT NOW AND GET OUT OF THE #%$&(&^%#@% CANOE."

Now I really had to get out, because it was the second time I'd called the canoe a bad name, and I knew it would be out to get me.

Eric paddled us to the shore without another word. I'm pretty sure he thought some, but he didn't say them. I got out, almost falling into the water and turning myself into a giant super-absorbent Tampax. He turned the canoe back around and continued on without me. This wasn't how I'd pictured it going down, but I knew I had better let him a) work out and b) work *me* out of his system. Looking like the Michelin man, I trudged back around the lake and beat him to the car by only half an hour.

By the time we'd loaded the canoe onto the top of our rental car and hopped in, we were well on our way back to our happy place. Yes, I know I don't deserve him. I don't question it; I just count my blessings.

That night we dined out—did I mention we were starving to death on broccoli and whole-wheat tabbouleh?—to celebrate our marriage. Eric had arranged for flowers to be delivered to our table before we got there. The aroma was scrumptious: cow, cooked cow! Yay! And, of course, the flowers. I looked at Eric's wind-chafed, sunburned face and almost melted from the heat of adoring him. Or maybe it was from the flame of the candle, which I was huddling over to stay warm. What was wrong with the people in this state? Somebody needed to buy Montana a giant heater. We held hands and traded swipes of Chapstick.

He interrupted my moment. "I have a confession to make. And I promise you are really going to think this is funny later."

Uh oh. "Spill it, baby."

"Remember when I paddled us toward the middle of the lake as hard as I could?"

"I'm trying to block the whole experience out of my mind."

"Yeah, well, let me tell you, sweetness, it was about ten times worse for me than you. But do you remember what you said about falling in, yadda yadda, frozen carcass next summer, blah blah?"

I didn't dignify this with an answer, but he didn't need one. "Well, you were in front of me, breathing into your paper bag or whatever, when I looked down, straight down, into the eyes and nostrils of a giant, bloated, frozen, very dead, fully intact, floating ELK CARCASS."

"You're lying."

"I am not. It was so close to the surface that if you hadn't still had those tears in your eyes, there is no way you wouldn't have seen it. You could have touched its head with your hand without even getting your wrist wet."

"No, you did **NOT** take me out on a lake with giant frozen dead animals floating in it." A macabre version of Alphabits cereal popped into my mind.

"Yes, I did," he said, and he hummed a few bars of Queen's "We are the Champions."

"Oh my God. If I had seen it right then, I would have come unhinged."   "More unhinged. I know. I was terrified you would capsize us and then you would quadruple freak out in the water bumping into that thing. I had to paddle for my life."

He was right. I let him enjoy *his* moment; I'm glad he confessed. But I will never canoe on a tundra lake with Eric again. Even if I got my courage up, he would never invite me. He couldn't have engineered a better moment to make me eager to get back in the pool, though.

POUTING ALL THE WAY

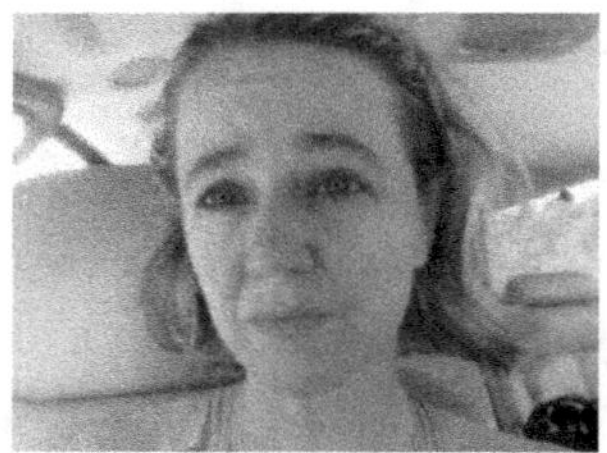

Above: Can you say "107 degrees?"

The word *endurance* defines my life. "Quitters never win and winners never quit" was the mantra of my childhood, thanks to my steely father. *Thanks, Dad!* I needed that for triathlon. Thank goodness Mom's mantra ("Are you really going to leave the house looking like that?") never quite stuck, or I'd never have gotten into those double-padded bike shorts.

Over the course of one hot August day, I did an Olympic-plus reverse triathlon. Lest you be too impressed, let me assure you that reversing the order of events in a triathlon makes a *huge* difference. Running with fresh, non-biked-out legs is much easier, and swimming after any high-temperature activity is nothing more than a great way to cool down. So, a run followed by a swim equals triathlon-training nirvana. Plus, getting to dash into the air-conditioned house and have conference calls with clients between "events" brought my heart rate down and gave me time to recharge.

But it was still a challenging day. I had postponed that morning's six a.m. run due to a headache, after having postponed last night's bike due to an ugly mood swing, and I knew I was facing a midday swim as well. I was under a big deadline on a project for a client, which I was managing to just barely get enough done on to make finishing on time possible but unpleasant. And my beloved and I, normally blissed-out and gaga, were shredding each other for no clear reason.

I set off alone for my 10K at 8:00 a.m., the Shuffle on as loud as I could stand without risking permanent hearing loss. I was jamming to Bon Jovi's "Runaway" with my black Tifosi sunglasses over my half-closed eyes. Within the first mile, I went from "I feel surprisingly good" to "WTF." Sprawled on my back, I tried to figure out how I could fall on flat pavement. I studied the road behind me and saw it: a rock—medium-sized, innocuous and apparently without a twinge of guilt, the rat bastard. For ten seconds I surveyed my middle-aged parts. Both hands and both knees were bleeding and painful, but I had no broken bones. My back was bleeding, too, from the automatic (but too-late) shoulder roll I had executed. I wiped off the gravel and a few angry "why make it so hard on me today, God" tears, and started running again.

At about the two-mile mark, I was cruising along the running path beside the concrete aquaduct that is Brays Bayou and cursing the sun when I realized I would not make it through the run without an emergency visit to the McDonald's bathroom. Oh, joy. I sprinted across the street for five minutes of fun getting in and out of sweaty spandex in a bathroom that had yet to be cleaned up from the weekend rush. A few more angry tears slipped out before I could stop them.

I started running again. The rest of the run was uncomfortable but required no more Britney Spears-like stops at public restrooms. I ran the specified distance at the specified pace (with a subtraction for the Mickey D's incident, because this was not a race, after all).

Next up: a one-hour break for a conference call with a prospective client about a proposal we had sent to them. I spent the last five minutes of the conference call with the phone on mute while I put together my water bottles, Nuun tablets, energy bars and GU, swim gear, and a sack lunch for Eric. As soon as I hung up, I made a dash for our pool, where I met Eric. I swam two thousand meters, which was a good bit more than Olympic distance; actually, it was even more than Half Ironman distance. My bronchitis from a few weeks before was finally abating, so I choked less than usual, but I choked nonetheless and struggled to keep my sucky attitude from getting worse.

Now I had to take another one-hour break to prepare and transmit draft documents to a different client. Finally, I hopped on the bike for a solo ride along the scenic, sweet-smelling (ha!) bayou in one-hundred-plus degree heat. It was a quick ride—about twenty-three miles in one and a half hours—because it's hard to get up any speed when you have to stop for traffic lights every mile or so. I managed not to crash, even when I dodged the clouds of little black bugs that I kept spitting out of my teeth. The sweat burned in my road rash from earlier.

And then I was done. I took stock of the day: I'd personally generated an entire load of laundry, my house was still dirty, I hadn't fed my kids, my husband, or the animals, and I would be working late to meet my deadline.

But I'd finished my triathlon training for the day with only minor injuries, and even my black toenail had survived intact. I was thankful for the chance to make up for flaking out the day before—if the kids weren't with their grandparents, my training would have been over before it started.

I was sure that I didn't crack a smile the entire time, though. I might even have pouted most of the way, and I shed tears more than once. I racked my brain for why this was fun—oh yeah, because I like to suffer—and why I still had cellulite. But I will say this: on days like this, I am a warrior goddess. I fight against traffic, smog, my job, my hormones, medium-sized rocks, the heat, sunscreen in my eyes, and my inner demons. I absolutely know that Dara Torres is not a fluke among over-forty women. We all have more in us than we use, and I think God was teaching me a lesson that day about stick-to-it-ness. A lesson I know I need for the really tough days—both in real life and in triathlon. Days like these remind me that I am not a quitter. I am an example to my children. I run the race to finish, not for speed. And somewhere along the way, I have become not just a woman spending quality time with her triathlete husband, but a real triathlete.

CREATURE FROM THE BLACK LAGOON

I have never been a swimmer. My girls are elite swimmers who spent hours every day in the pool at the peak of their racing. My husband is a swimmer who absolutely loves to swim. I swim as a means to an end; one cannot triathlon without completing the swim portion of the race. But I approach swimming as a "just the minimum, just in time" element of my training.

If I didn't have to get wet and wear a bathing suit, swimming would be fine. No, that's a lie. I also don't like getting water in my ears, I hate being cold, and I abhor the smell of chlorine that won't come out of my pores with just one shower. But what I hate most is dark water.

My first triathlons were in the Caribbean Sea; the warm, clear, crystalline Caribbean Sea. The first time I swam in open water sans snorkel was in Cane Bay on St. Croix. My swim buddy Theresa and I got stuck over a barely-submerged reef littered with sea urchins and had to fingertip-walk our way out, getting stung over and over again by tiny jellyfish. But it wasn't scary, it was an adventure in a magical world. Just after we made it over the reef, a pod of dolphins swam under us, which I interpreted as God and Mother Nature's blessing.

But when it comes to dark water, I am permanently moored on *Creature from the Black Lagoon*. I've had several occasions to relive that horror: learning to ski on a lake as a child, canoeing on that ice-lined lake on my honeymoon.

We were four months away from the Half Ironman when my step-daughter Marie invited us to swim in her gym's quarry lake, where many local triathletes train for open water swimming. My phobic hatred of dark water kicked in full force.

Every step I took towards that beautiful yet dark quarry lake deepened my fear, and the swim itself didn't start well. As soon as I was in the water, I felt something bite me in the vicinity of my diaphragm, not once, but twice. I squealed and shot up out of the water, stripping off my swimsuit. Eric held a towel around me on the dock while I searched for the vicious insects. I found a small twig in the chest area, but no bugs. There were only two tiny red welts on my chest. Where the hell had the gigantic water creature that stung me gone? This was not the work of any mere twig.

I glanced at my chest again, and the welts had disappeared. OK, maybe it was a twig. Or a figment of my imagination. I sat on the dock wearing nothing but a towel and stared at the water, oblivious to the swimmers getting in and out of the water.

"Do you want to wait for me here on the dock?" Eric asked. He was shooting for gracious, but he was not about to give up his swim to my hysteria.

"Yes," I sniffed.

Before I could say another word to him—like "please help me back into my suit so I don't have to sit here naked with strangers"—he was in the water and swimming freestyle toward the first buoy. Twelve minutes later, he finished his first lap of the course. By this point, there were six men on the dock with me, as I sat with my bathing suit in my lap.

Before he began his second lap, Eric stopped. "Do you need anything?"

"What? You mean something like not to be sitting here buck naked with six strangers?" My facial expression matched the dulcet tone of my voice.

He got out without a word (now he was the one who was scared), and we found some bushes and got me re-dressed in semi-privacy. I decided to try again.

Back into the lake we went. I put my face in the water, and it was like a vise clamped my lungs shut. The water was an impenetrable green forest. The feeling of its immensity around me was too much. I made it blindly to the first buoy. The best I can say of my performance is that my aim was better than I thought it would be. Other than that, I was two deep breaths from falling apart.

I made it to the second buoy. I kept thinking it would get easier, but the farther I got from the shore, the worse it became. I started hyperventilating, and my heart was trying to jackhammer its way out of my chest.

Halfway to buoy three, I was sobbing, which, along with hyperventilation, cuts into one's effectiveness as a swimmer. The long-suffering Eric joined me as I cut straight through the center of the course for the dock. I swam sidestroke the whole way so I could sight the shore.

It was completely demoralizing. My swimming had improved greatly over the last four months' training in a pool. I had three open-water ocean triathlons under my belt. To think that I might be unable to finish the lake swim in my upcoming Half Ironman because of the terrors was awful, so Eric and I brainstormed solutions.

First, I suggested, maybe being in the water with 2,500 people rather than one would decrease the feeling of immensity of the lake around me. Next, Eric suggested we drive to lakes within an hour or two of Houston each Sunday for the next six weeks and practice—I'd just keep getting *in* lakes and getting back out alive. Lastly, I planned to go back to the pool and swim 1820 meters doing sidestroke. If I could swim the full distance sidestroke within the allotted seventy-five minutes, I could stare at the sky and shore rather than put my face into black water. As a last resort only, of course.

I had four months left to worry about it.

THE STORM

That summer, I was trying to balance childrearing, my career, my new marriage, and the symptoms of perimenopause, and it felt like climbing Mount Everest in a blizzard with a backpack full of lead. I wanted Eric to understand what I was going through. I wanted to make him understand the storm of my despair when I was buffeted by life and hormones, and how I felt after the storm passed.

I knew that it didn't seem like there was much in the world for me to despair over in the first place, but there I was, swinging back and forth between sunshine and thunderstorms, euphoria and anguish, ability and disability. How could two opposing conditions occupy one small place almost simultaneously? But everyone's seen the sun shine when it rains.

Most days I am known for radiating sunshine, but sometimes it storms. The night came that I was out of town on a business trip, sitting in a nondescript hotel room in nondescript nowhere with tears raining down my face as the rain fell outside. We'd just had a mighty fight because he had failed to update me on something material about one of our kids, something I took as an intentional omission and treated as such, and something he claimed he just forgot. I was empty, spent, wasted. I learned early in life that appearance is not just important, it is everything. It is bad manners and self-indulgent self-pity to show others that ugly stormy stuff, so I put the "clear skies" face on for the world. But I don't have to for Eric.

The ultimate compliment of our closeness as a couple, of our connection, is that my private world includes him now. I don't hide from him, and he is not afraid of my moods. He knows them and can handle them like no one else.

I wanted so badly to keep my husband out of these storms, and I used to run away from him when they came, trying to protect him from me. But he wanted to show me he is strong enough to protect us both. I hope he's right, because he'll have plenty of chances to show it.

Inside my head that night there was an electrical storm. I couldn't hear myself think for all the noise it was making; I couldn't think clearly at all. The thunder rolled deep into the center of me and settled there, burning me from the inside out. Not like a lightning strike, but like a slow building burn, like getting into a bathtub that is just a little too hot at first and realizing five minutes later that the heat is suffocating you. The heaviness in my core was pulling me down by the back of my neck and folding my body into the fetal position. I was a hot mess, and not in a good way.

My anger strikes like lightning. Most of the time, the flashes are internal, but sometimes they flash out as well. As confusion and anger take over, I give in, telling myself that next time I have to fight harder, because it is wrong to be so weak and hurt myself and hurt my husband. But who can stop the weather?

And then we are caught in a wild storm, irrational and unpredictable. You can rage at it, but it has to run its course. When it's over in me and I am depleted, Eric has become the storm. He has to jab and thrust, and I'm the only one around to take the blows. It's only fair.

And it was, for me. Over. I was limp and beaten, and, what's more, I was wrong and knew it. Why had I jumped to the conclusion that my husband was deceptive with me, and had intentionally hidden something about one of the kids? It wasn't rational. He had never deceived me before. Now that the storm inside me had passed, I couldn't find any part of me that really believed he was dishonest. What the hell was wrong with me?

I would be angry at me if I were him, too. Yet, as bad as I felt, of one thing I was sure: if the storm came again, I would be just as powerless to stop it. Werewolf, storm, whatever it was called, I was absolutely terrified of next time.

DING DONG, IS THE WEREWOLF DEAD?

Each month during the first ten weeks of my five-month training plan, I would transform into the rabid werewolf beast. In addition to the psychotic rages and crippling migraines that only came with the moon, some changes were permanent, like heavy ridges in my once-smooth fingernails, dilated pupils, and a weight gain that had crept up to twenty-five pounds over the year I had experienced perimenopause, or whatever the hell it was. We were all scared of me, and as the triathlon training ratcheted up in intensity, I questioned whether I would make it to the end.

My mother approached very carefully one day. She called from a safe distance, "Have you tried Dr. Hotze {Hotze Health and Wellness Center, http://www.hotzehwc.com}? I have friends who say he's saved women's lives when they had nowhere else to turn."

"Never heard of him," I said.

"He does some kind of hormone thing. He has a radio show. And he's in Houston."

I would have tried anything at this point, which I guess makes me one of those women who had nowhere else to turn. And he was in Houston, where I lived. But he didn't take insurance, and he was expensive.

"You're worth it. We're worth it. At least try," my husband said. God bless Eric.

So I did. The doctor at the Hotze Health and Wellness Center listened carefully to my tale of woe. "The only way you gained twenty-five pounds in six months without a hormonal issue or some other medical issue is if you laid in bed stuffing Tootsie Rolls in your mouth the whole time," he said. God bless him, too.

When he told me I was not insane, I cried. I couldn't help it. I begged for help, and he promised me that he and his staff could deliver. He had seen hundreds of women just like me, albeit not all as severe. He said that in his opinion, fibromyalgia was often a symptom of some other problem, so hearing that I felt like I had fibromyalgia made sense. The symptoms I was experiencing were fibromyalgic, and given the other factors, indicators of a severe hormonal imbalance.

He prescribed bioidentical hormones—nonsynthetic, natural hormones—and a yeast-elimination diet. He explained that my primary issue was an overabundance of estrogen; he called me "estrogen dominant." Wow. Most people that know me would agree with that without any medical explanation.

He cringed when I told him that my gyno had prescribed birth control pills for my symptoms.

"The hormone in that birth control is estrogen. She just pumped you full of more of what was already poisoning you."

Interesting word, poison. Because that's one way I'd described how I felt. Like I was poisoned.

"Time will tell if you are in perimenopause, but it sure sounds likely, even given your relatively young age. But the treatment for perimenopause is to address the symptoms, so it doesn't really matter, anyway," he explained.

He prescribed progesterone, which would address the long psychotic stretches and the migraines. He added cortisol for my constant state of stress (dilated pupils, anxiety, sleeplessness). He put me on testosterone to boost my energy. And he gave me thyroid to nudge me further into balance and address my ridged nails and ice-cold hands and feet. He also provided nystatin to kill off the yeast in my digestive tract in conjunction with a three-month-long diet adjustment.

In four days, I felt fifty percent better. In eight days, I had lost eleven pounds. In two weeks, I wondered if I'd really felt as bad as I remembered. In one month, I was me again. For real. No exaggeration. They gave me my life back.

They gave me my inner athlete back, too. Hell, yeah. 70.3, here we come. The werewolf is dead, and nobody misses her.

IT'S A LOT LIKE A HEART ATTACK.

When a forty-something woman is preparing for an endurance event, every single minute of training is urgent. Day-to-day fitness is important all the time, but it's a long-term investment without short-term urgency. Ramping up for an endurance race requires a strict regimen in the short term; it's definitely urgent. Urgent like a trip to the emergency room for a heart attack. If you knew that unless you zoomed to the hospital by ambulance right now you would die before nightfall of a heart attack, you'd clear your schedule and jump onboard, wouldn't you? That's how the middle-aged (non)athlete has to approach endurance training.

But in the real world, shit happens. Emergencies crap all over your training schedule. You get the flu. Your kids have swim meets, debate tournaments, and choir concerts. Dogs lose their eyes {All of these are actual events that occurred during race prep for Eric and me, at one time or another}. What, that hasn't happened at your house? For our Longhorn Half Ironman, we had to work around my uncontrolled hormones, three kids and their activities, Eric's travel to India {He literally took his bicycle and a forty-pound training stand with him.} and a hurricane in Houston. Yet every workout on the schedule leading up to your [marathon, Half Ironman, century ride, ultramarathon, ocean swim, Ironman] is there for a reason. Fit it in, make it up, or risk death on the course. OK, maybe what you risk is just failure, but death is an outside possibility if you push too hard with too little training.

I'm slightly less of a stickler than Eric, who won't even consider doing an event if he misses more than five percent of the training. But if he scratches, I scratch, so in the end it's all the same. Since I know this about him, and I balance it against my absolute abhorrence of wasted money on entrance fees, training is that much more important to me. Damn straight, it's like a heart attack.

Now that sets the priority level for training, but it doesn't solve the multitask/sacrifice puzzle. Somehow, most of the time, we make the pieces fit. Eric and I treat training as date time. We work out together ninety percent of the time, and we make it fun, riding in great places like Brazos Bend State Park, making playlists for each other's Shuffles (Sean Paul!), and grabbing a meal afterwards at Barnaby's Café. We hold hands on our side-by-side trainers as we watch *Friday Night Lights* on Netflix. I've patted his cute behind a time or two on our runs.

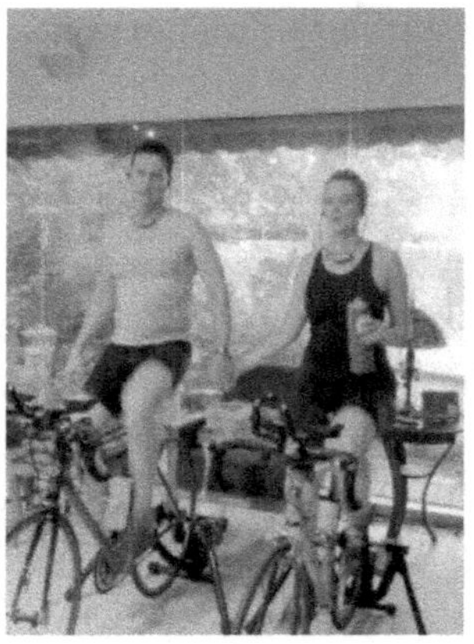

We cut out lunches and coffee breaks in favor of eating in the car on the way back from a noon swim. We've kissed our kids goodbye at swim meet warm-ups and sprinted out the door for a run, making it back in time to catch half the meet. Half is better than nothing, and we've noticed that most of the parents drop off and don't come back at all, so we not only beat the pack but our kids think we're rock stars.

And it certainly doesn't suck to hear them telling their friends about their crazy athletic parents with pride in their voices.

We don't watch TV. We don't luxuriate over the Sunday paper. There are no long baths. I don't chitchat on the phone with my mom unless I'm driving— and only with a headset! I promise! All those activities can wait until the week after race day. Before the race, while we train, training is a heart attack, and any fat we can find gets sliced right out with a sharp scalpel.

As a result, we don't schedule back-to-back races. (Anymore— after a one-month stretch of weekly distance bike races and half marathons nearly cost our sanity, we got smarter.) Life requires breathers and catch-up time for doing doctors' visits and orthodontists' appointments and grocery shopping and trips to buy graphing calculators. But while we're standing in line at Old Navy with a teenager and a semester's worth of new blue jeans, our bodies appreciate the time to rejuvenate and heal.

And sometimes we just have to say no. No, I won't chair the canned food drive this month, but I can in the spring. No, I won't put together a department video for the holiday party in my spare time. (Ever). Other times, it's ourselves and the race we have to say no to. As in, No, I just can't fit in the training that race requires. Let's look for a different one, at a different time.

And that's OK. Because even though endurance event training is a lot like a heart attack, it has a critical difference from the real thing: I can always cancel a race, but I don't get that choice with a heart attack.

Until then, though, you can be sure I'm following that schedule unless someone has defibrillator shock paddles against my chest.

LONGHORN DREAMIN'

The last two weeks before the Longhorn 70.3 was for healing. We began to taper down our daily training from an average of three hours of training down to two, down to one, to let our bodies recover from the little aches, pains, and strains so we could make our peak performances on race day. My main ouchy after eighteen weeks of training was iliotibial band syndrome (ITBS) in my left knee and thigh. When I asked my orthopedist how to heal it, he said, "No more running. Then on race day, run like mad." I was relegated to aqua-jogging until the big event.

We would have had a little more free time with the taper-down, but Hurricane Ike had knocked out the power a couple of weeks before, and we were still driving an hour round-trip to a different pool every day. That was disappointing, but workable.

I'd done such a good job at fueling that, while I was as fit as I have ever been in my life, I didn't look as thin as I'd hoped. Don't get me wrong. All my skinny clothes were a little too big, but I knew I'd look curvy and plump next to the competitive triathletes. Eric said I looked like Madonna. Ha! But I no longer had the upper body that earned me the nickname "Noodle" in high school. There's nothing like being married to a very lean man to motivate a woman, for real. Eric had to fight not to lose any more weight, and the threat of me going out and buying him 32 pants and throwing out his 34s was good inspiration.

My only real *ugh* was that we'd trained as a team but we would race alone. The triathlon started in waves by gender and age, so we wouldn't start together, and even if we did, we'd lose each other in the water. No Eric to encourage me, or caution me, or smile at me, or for me to focus on instead of obsessing about my own darn self. I hated that. It was Han Solo time: more than six and a half hours with just me and my brain and body.

With nine days to go, I was dreaming about the race all the time, kind of like the recurring dream I had in college and law school, where I skipped class all semester and showed up naked to take the final. Only this time, I show up naked on race day and I don't know how to change a flat. Or I brought the wrong fuel. Or I'm missing my Butt Butter in the transition area. Or I freak out and hyperventilate in the middle of the lake. Those kinds of things.

But I knew I was ready. Eric had coached me on the swim and bike big time, and he believed in me.

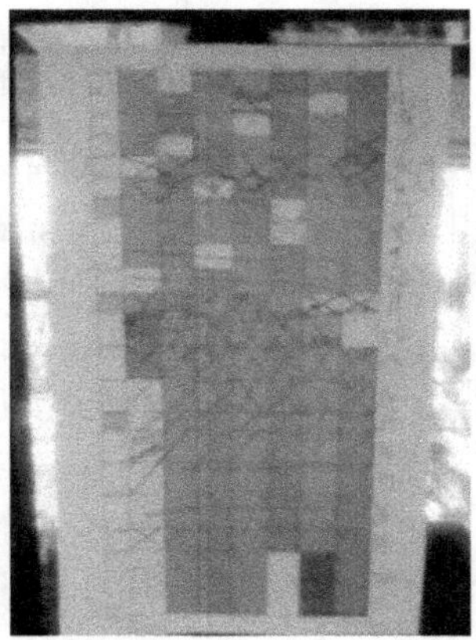

Six months before the race, I was in bed most of the time, not sure how I was going to cope with how bad I had felt for so long. Then my clever husband challenged me to this triathlon, giving me a goal that cattle-prodded me into fighting back against my hormones and returning to life. It was almost show time.

THE TRIUMPH OF MIND OVER MATTER

By the Saturday before the Sunday race, I had made myself ill with nerves. I tried to focus on how far I had come and that I was ready, instead of how intimidated I was by the magnitude of the event.

In 20 weeks, I had forced myself to become a swimmer, one who could swim for well over a mile at a respectable pace without stopping. I could ride a bicycle 18 miles an hour for over 100 miles. I could comfortably run a half marathon. A very small percentage of the people in the world can do these things. I knew this. I knew how far I had come, from zero to here in 20 weeks. Regardless of how I did in the race, time-wise, I had nearly accomplished my goal. I had faced the hardest part of the challenge and beat it already.

But I still had to complete the race, along with 2,499 other competitors, the majority of whom would do it faster than me.

We got to Austin and went to the athletes' village to pick up the race packet, and it was SOOOOO intimidating. The people there all looked like they had just stepped out of *Triathlete* magazine, which many of them had. We passed by Michellie Jones and our daughter Liz said, "Hey, I've got a picture of that woman up on my door!" It was an ad out of *Triathlete*.

We also had to get out and do our final nerve-calming workout. It was ninety-one degrees and dusty at the course, but oh how amazing.

Imagine the setup required for 2,500 athletes: bandstands, food stands, medical tents, and racks for the 2,500 bikes that had to be left overnight. Security was high; I thought our carbon-fiber bikes were nice, but they were mere Chevrolets compared to the line-up of Mercedes and Rolls Royces.

The water was seventy-eight degrees—wetsuit legal—but when we got in the lake I wasn't cold, so I opted against the claustrophobic suit. The water was clear enough that I could see the ends of my fingers while swimming, which may not sound like much for freaky me, but it was OK. The smell was good, and the taste wasn't bad. I didn't like how my hands got tangled in the weeds as we swam through the shallows, but we swam out to a few buoys and I didn't implode. A miracle.

We got to bed early, and then it was 5:00 a.m. and time to rock and roll. The first trial of the event was getting there. We had to park offsite, stand in long lines, and shuttle in. In fact, they had to push the start time back by half an hour because shuttling went so slowly. This allowed for full daylight at the start, which was great, but meant we finished when it was hotter, which was brutal.

After braving the long porta-potty lines, we stood still for our numbers and ages to be written all over us with Sharpies. The age mark was great, because it allowed me to see who I was passing that counted in my age group, and who was passing me. Then we set up our transition areas, hooking our bicycles onto our allotted space on the long rows of metal bars, and lining our accoutrements up on a towel: race number belts, bike shoes, helmets, sunglasses, moleskin ankle patches, water bottles, running shoes, socks, and extra GUs. I put my baggy of ibuprofen, Excedrin, and Afrin, plus four GUs and a Bumble Bar for energy into the bento bag on my bike. I grabbed my goggles, ear wax, and swim cap, began to stretch, and breathed deeply.

Eric and I were able to stand together until five minutes before the start. As I moved away from him, numb with fear, I kept looking back at him for reassurance. The pros would start first, then the thirty- to thirty-five-year-old guys, then my "geezer" group of forty- to forty-five-year-old women. Eric's wave would start a full thirty minutes behind mine; mine was to be five minutes behind the pros.

Each group wore different-colored swim caps. Me and my old lady peeps wore pearl pink, which matched my tri suit ensemble. I entered the water to make my way to the neck-deep starting position.

And then it was go time. I was in my first Half Ironman, swimming in a cold dark lake without my husband. The swim was *very* physical. Even in my geriatric wave, there were a lot of body collisions. By the first buoy I was so panicked that I was hyperventilating —my biggest fear—and had stopped and almost bailed out.

A nice woman stopped with me and asked, "Are you OK?"

"I will be, I just have to get myself under control," I replied, treading water.

It felt like an eternity, but it was probably only ten seconds later when I realized I could swim on my back until I could breathe, go wide out of the flailing traffic, and then just roll back over and do it. I could not throw it all away in the first five minutes. So I restarted. My new guardian angel wouldn't leave me until I was swimming solidly; I wish I knew who she was so I could have thanked her later.

The swim got harder as the next wave's faster swimmers started catching up with us, and we started catching the slowest swimmers of the wave in front of us. Suddenly there were hundreds of people in the middle of the lake, kicking, whacking, and all jacked up on adrenaline. A guy walloped me once and then decided to pass under me, shoving my body up out of the water. I literally whaled back and slugged him. This might not have been the smartest or right thing to do, but he didn't even pause. I put the werewolf back in her cage and kept swimming.

I had minor navigational difficulties, but I made it, I **made** it, I *really really really* **made it** all the way through that violent lake swim. When I got out of the water to start the uphill run towards my bike, my thirteen-year-old son Clark was waiting for me in the spectators' area. That sweet boy ran beside me on the other side of the fence and slapped me a high-five. I teared up but tamped the emotion back down and stayed focused.

I went through transition methodically, chanting, "GU, moleskin, sunglasses," then ran the hundred yards with my bike to the place where we could mount. My parents and my eleven-year-old daughter Susanne were right there, cheering me on. I cheered back.

The bike is the fun part. I love my pink Trek Pilot 5.2 WSD. I love the feel of the air on my face, hitting forty miles an hour down a good hill with the wind at my back. I love cornering. I love everything but the super-painful bike seat. But that day, I didn't even notice my ouchy nether regions. The bike segment went really well for me. My first hour I averaged 19 miles per hour, and I finished with a 17.7 miles per hour average. I managed to choke down an energy bar, I remembered to GU, I drank twelve ounces an hour, I took my Advil thirty minutes before the finish, and I backed off progressively over the last hour to give my legs recovery time for the run. Thanks, coach!

I got off the bike on schedule for my original overall goal time of 6:30, but there was one small problem: this run was going to be a death march. Due to ITBS, I hadn't run in six weeks. I had readjusted my goal time to seven hours for the whole triathlon as a result.

My family was at transition again, cheering me on. I managed a fist pump then, but I knew by the time I finished the first mile that I was in trouble. There was absolutely no spring or lift in my step. Apparently, to run well, you should actually *run* when you're training. Aqua-jogging was better than nothing, but is no substitute for the real thing. My feet felt like bleeding stumps. And when we got out on the black asphalt, oh boy, it was mega hills and waves of heat.

In mile two, I was thinking again about bailing out. Forget finishing by my revised goal time; I needed a new strategy for how to finish by the eight-hour cut-off. My first idea? *Screw strategy, fake an injury and get off this burning asphalt hell.* But that thought was fleeting. I had made a big investment to get to where I was, and I, by golly, was going to finish. So I decided to run the flats and downhills (run? I'm not sure you could call it that. Plod, trot, shuffle, hobble?) and walk up.

As I finished mile three, I met Eric coming the other direction and we slapped hands. I did a quick calculation and broke into my first smile in hours. Eric was going to close our thirty-minute start gap and catch me.

When I hit the halfway point at 6.55 miles, I began to believe I had it licked. I told myself, *It's just a 10K, you can do this. It's like running out to Fondren Middle School and back. You do that all the time.* (Of course, those runs left out the hills, the 1.2-mile swim-brawl, and the 56-mile bike). My pace picked up a smidge. Eric was a few minutes closer when we passed each other again.

I made it to the ten-mile mark. Now I knew I was going to finish, but I was in almost too much pain to care. I had never hurt that bad in my life, not in natural childbirth, not with gall bladder or heart surgery (a long story for another time). If it had been a training run, I would have quit. But quitting was not an option that day.

I could see Eric over my shoulder. At mile 12.75, he kicked in a last spurt and caught up with me. I didn't even have the energy to bawl. We held hands and walked the last hill. At thirteen miles, the hill ended, the course entered the finishing chute, and we ran the last tenth of a mile together, with Clark running beside us outside the fence. Eric and I finished together, with times of 6:23 and 6:53, respectively. Slower than we'd liked, but acceptable given the heat.

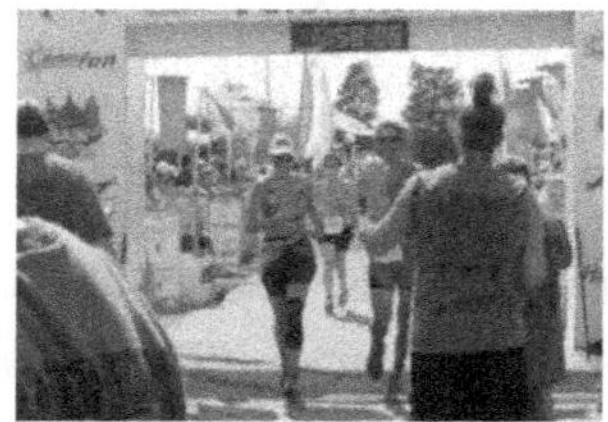

Clark pulled up chairs for us and took off our shoes. "It's a good thing you didn't have to crawl across the finish like a guy did a half hour ago."

Crawling was an option? I should have crawled.

Susanne sponged my face. Eric's daughters were there now, too, and Liz dreamed aloud about doing a triathlon herself, while Marie tried not to let us get her sweaty. My dad fired questions about the course, and my mom fussed and clucked.

It was an agony of true pain and exhaustion, but that only heightened my sense of accomplishment. I totally dug the long-sleeved wicking t-shirt they gave us. Truly, it was one of the most perfect moments of my life. And to cross the finish line with Eric, a finish line that represented so much more than just a race, meant the world to me. To be met by the people I loved most in the world? Amazing. Take that, estrogen!

But only a few hours after the race, I didn't feel at peace and satisfied with my efforts anymore. Neither did Eric. We were obsessed with analyzing what we had done wrong and what we could do better the next time. There was nothing in the whole world I wanted more than a do-over—as soon as possible.

That race, as awesome as it was, was not the conclusion I had thought it would be. That race was the beginning. The beginning of something powerful and uncontrollable, a new beast in my breast. Something monstrous to rival my werewolf hormones for domination. Something that didn't acknowledge pain, injury, illness, or real life. Something that I wasn't sure then and am not sure now is a particularly good thing, but it had me by the throat, my eyes were bulging, and I wasn't even trying to break free of the chokehold.

By midnight of that same day, we had registered for the Conroe Iron Star triathlon, only one month away.

SCRATCH

When the alarm went off the morning after the Longhorn 70.3, Eric and I were euphoric. We should have been exhausted. We'd flown from Austin to Orlando after our big race and stayed up late to register for the next one. It had been a long day and a short night, and Eric had to give a presentation at a conference in a couple of hours. I had tagged along as the trailing spouse, and I planned to make the most of it. I jumped out of bed, sleepy but eager—until I took my first step.

"Holy Mother Goose and Grimm," I yelped, and sank to the floor. My left leg hurt like a sumbitch, and it didn't want to play rise-and-shine just yet.

"Whassamatta," Eric said into his pillow.

I didn't answer. He rolled over and got up. "Wow, I'm a little stiff," he said.

My brain was too tired to think of the right foul name to call my beloved. I tried to walk again. I was able to, but just. "I'm a little stiff, too," I lied.

Somehow I made it through the Orlando trip, hobbling through the hotel and groaning a lot. I was happy to get back on a plane to Houston three days later so that I could be miserable in my own space.

A few weeks, several massages, lots of stretching, multiple visits to the physical therapist, and countless hours in hot baths later, I tried running. Nothing doing: my ITBS was much worse.

Under matrimonial and medical advice, and even as I protested that "Yes, I *can* do this," I listened to the rational rather than the emotional side of my brain for once and sat out the Conroe Iron Star Half Ironman. While with rehab and therapy I'd kept training, I was not healed yet. This race was just not special enough to jeopardize our training for the event I really wanted to do, which was a marathon on our anniversary. What says "I love you and I'm so glad I married you" better than 26.1 miles over concrete at 7:00 a.m. on New Year's Day?

The war in my head had raged over this decision for weeks. Childhood slogans haunted my mind: "Don't be a quitter!" and "Mind over matter!" I felt so guilty knowing that if I opted out, Eric would too. Probably only because it was me, not him, Eric was clear-headed about this (yep, that was a dig) and laid out the scenarios of me either a) setting the training for the marathon back by overdoing it in Conroe, or b) having a big physical and emotional blowout on the run and never doing another triathlon again in my life. He was more scared of b.

I mourned the big decision by gorging on Wingstop after an hour-long swim. Anyway, paradoxically this now meant I needed to add more running to my schedule and probably take out one day of bicycling for a few months. I was advised to hold my pace to a short-strided trot, but that for one short run each week I could do a few repetitions of striding out for a couple hundred yards, then decelerate. When I could do one run a week at a decent pace without significant pain, I could take the brakes off.

So we spent three hundred dollars on the race and didn't even get the t-shirts. Being mature about this really sucked.

DRIVEN

To say that I am driven is an understatement. I know how hard this is on my loved ones, and I am blessed that my husband finds this overachiever urge a positive. Some people have labeled me Little Miss Perfect, and others have cheered my failures as much as my successes. I understand. I may not like it, but I understand.

This aspect of my personality was a tremendous problem in my first marriage, at which I failed, and I'm sure I don't have to explain how much I hate to fail. It absolutely ate me up that I had to scratch on the Conroe Half Ironman.

The intensity of my drive has prevented friendships and cost me friendships. Even when I am not competing with others, I am driving myself hard enough that most people don't want to be close to me. I don't push the people around me to be my clones, but they feel my internal pressure.

It's hard for me to relax, because I don't do downtime well. I understand that some people enjoy watching TV, but I can't, unless I'm multitasking. I used to read books; I don't any more. I do have a nasty Facebook addiction, but nobody's perfect.

Does it help those who can't stand the constant barrage of events and contests to know that the person most damaged by all the pressure is me? Probably not. But I do tear myself into small pieces, over small things, fairly frequently. And I know I am not ever going to change.

I have some ugly memories of turning on myself, from ripping up second-place ribbons at a ninth-grade track meet, to cutting a dress into tiny pieces when it didn't fit me at the age of twenty-four. I wish I were kidding, and I wish I had that black dress with the little pearls all over it back now. I used to drink myself into a brainless heap so I wouldn't think about how I wasn't currently meeting my own exacting standards. I don't have that anesthetic anymore.

My drive is what makes me get up off the couch and put down my Cinnabon, then do a Half Ironman twenty weeks later. I create spreadsheets with plans and interim goals and deadlines, and determinedly cross off the days as I hit each mark. I'm wicked intense with a budget, too.

So it is with sheepish self-awareness and great personal satisfaction that I tell the world about a bike race that went really well for me. Working together, Eric and I won it. Not age group, not gender, but the whole race itself. It was only thirty-two miles, and it had only about a hundred entrants, but this represented a quantum leap from where I was last spring, and I was elated about it.

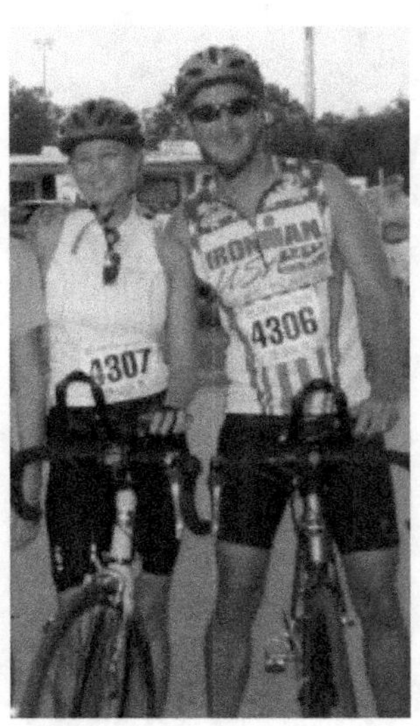

I want to achieve my best by doing hard work. Most days, just overcoming my hormonal desire to lick my wounds in a dark corner is an accomplishment. Some days I will come in last, but I want to give it my all in training and racing. I know that in this bicycle race, I did.

Why all that upfront self-analysis and confession, just to tell you about a podunk bike race? Because I feel guilty talking about these things. I don't want to make people who don't share my penchant for self-punishment think that my choices are a judgment on their lifestyles. I want my loved ones to know that this gift is a curse. But the force of my will allows me to take my mediocre talent to the modest levels of achievement necessary for me to maintain my sense of self.

It ain't all pretty, but it's me.

IT WAS A ROCKY RACCOON.

One fine Saturday morning during marathon training, Eric and I, feeling only moderate guilt, dropped the kids at their various events at 7:00 a.m. with promises to pick them up by two. Then we sped the one and a half hours north to Huntsville State Park to try out their dirt trails for our scheduled fifteen-mile run. We'd run on dirt before, but never on true trails. We were pumped for the adventure.

Unbeknownst to us, it was the day that six hundred runners were competing in the Rocky Raccoon 25K and 50K trail races. We got there just as the elite 50K runners were finishing the first of their two laps, so we ran our 25K with them. A 50K (31 miles) is considered a baby ultramarathon; longer than a traditional 26.1-mile marathon, but not by a heck of a lot. This was an impressive group and event.

Soon we blended into the super-supportive pack of colleagues-in-suffering, and the other runners started cheering us on, too. I sort of felt bad, because we a) weren't doing the whole race and b) were on our first lap while they were all on their second. We gave thumbs-ups and pumped our fists in the air, though, and joined the praise and encouragement bandwagon.

I want to be a trail runner when I grow up. Racing with those athletes gave me a new and profound respect for trail runners. We were constantly, and I mean constantly, scampering either up or down a hill, and I don't know which was worse. There were long patches of deep sand, and Eric and I fell several times on tree roots that were covered by leaves and pine needles—but most of the other runners had earth on their chests and back, too. Everybody just popped back up and kept limping along.

Because it is a long loop, you have to carry your hydration and fuel with you. We weren't prepared for that, so I had stuck GUs in my tights. Not so much fun. The race had some aid stations, but we didn't think it was right to use them since we hadn't paid an entrance fee. We did, however, seek and receive permission before we joined the runners, because it was too late to enter officially, so I did the 25K Rocky Raccoon and didn't get the t-shirt. Race shirt whore that I am, that bites.

I was wearing, for the second time, my new neutral Adidas Adistars and custom orthotics, which helped my knee. But at about the halfway point on that uneven terrain, my right hip and ankle started screaming for an ice pack and two Aleve.

The park and trails were beautiful, for a run, a hike, or a stationary meditation. There's a lake with a lot of marshy, swampy (in a good way) tributaries. It's mostly piney woods. We saw birds, alligators, and deer, and Eric had his first up close and personal meeting with a very alarmed armadillo. We ran over creaky wooden bridges across gullies and creeks and through marshy lowlands. Total coolness.

The trail's effect on our speed was enough that I shall not tell you how long it took us to run the distance. Suffice it to say that while we run much, much faster on the flat, we'd never run happier.

HAPPY ANNIVERSARY, BABY

Eric and I started the new year right, by celebrating our anniversary and running our first marathon. Well, the marathon prevented much celebrating before or after, but we felt celebratory, anyway.

The Texas Marathon was held on New Year's Day in Kingwood, north of Houston. Since that day was its tenth anniversary—happy anniversary to all of us!—the race bags and awards were outrageously good. We love our long-sleeved tees and giant bling longhorn-head medals.

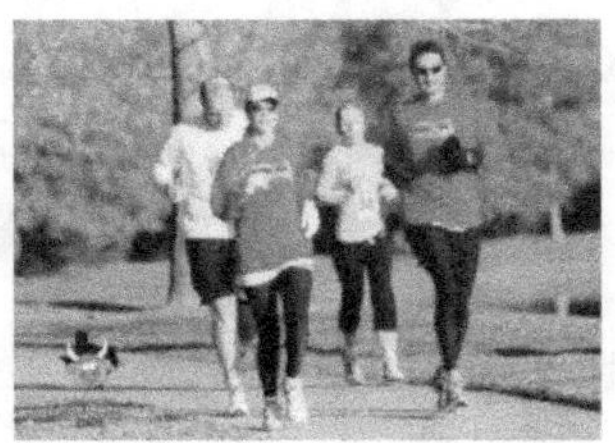

The 26.2-mile race curved around Lake Houston along narrow, heavily wooded greenbelt trails. It began at sunrise and was comprised of four circuits of a 6.55-mile loop. This was great, because we made it easily through the first three loops and were well into the fourth before we hit the famed 20-mile wall and lost all desire to

finish (or remain upright and alive).There was no way to bail out at that point, and I turned into a blubbering idiot. I barely finished.

"One step at a time, Pamela, you can do it," Eric urged.

And I did. We were pleased with our performances, especially because icy roads in December had cost us most of our last weeks of training. But we had promised to stay together and finish, even if we had to walk. We would stop for nothing but protruding broken bones or acute medical emergencies.

That day my blisters got blisters, I lost one of my black toenails, and I learned that Butt Butter ain't just for biking. But we stayed together and finished within three minutes of our goal time of five hours, and ended the day watching Cardinal football. I started the new year with my beloved and a checkmark next to one of my biggest life goals, and it was way easier than a Half Ironman. Awesomesauce.

AN OLD DOGTOR LEARNS NEW TRICKS

My father, AKA Dr. Dad, was raised up as a physician in the latter half of the twentieth century in a medical industry largely funded and influenced by pharmaceutical companies. He was taught, to a great degree, to prescribe pharmaceutical medicines; to focus on the problem, rather than prevention of the problem. He was not instructed much on wellness, vitamins, minerals, or the benefits of optimal nutrition. He sought this information out himself.

During his years as a doctor, he explored many alternatives to pharmaceuticals. Having had eight—yes, eight—back surgeries, he tried magnet therapy and inversion (the torture-rack booted devices where you hang upside down), and exercised religiously (a value he passed on to us kids). He constantly explored new diets and supplements. Meanwhile, he continued a fairly traditional private practice, focusing on the field of occupational medicine.

But in 2008, my hormonal issues introduced Dr. Dad to a whole new area of medicine: the use of bioidentical, non-synthetic, non-pharmaceutical, natural hormones, combined with a robust vitamin and mineral regimen and a yeast-free diet, to achieve optimal health and wellness. At the age of sixty-one, my father was born again.

He had watched with frustration as his aging father's health declined despite an overwhelming regimen of pharmaceuticals.

Some of those medicines were absolutely necessary, but others? Hard to say. His father's days kept getting shorter. He ate less. He was confused, and he was clumsy. These things are normal for a ninety-year-old man, but Dr. Dad asked himself if things really had to be that bad.

Dr. Dad was convinced that he should be treating the symptoms of the patient, not the numerical test values that fit into some range of normality for the population at large. He approached some of his father's issues with this belief and his newfound knowledge. Grandfather appeared to be hypothyroid, despite being nearly anorexic and having normal thyroid numbers. So Dr. Dad treated him with natural, bioidentical thyroid. He rubbed topical testosterone into the smooth skin inside his father's forearm. He supplemented his dad's diet with tiny amounts of iodine. And his father improved. Rapidly, markedly, and obviously, he got better. He ate more, he was awake longer, he gained weight, his skin took on a healthier hue, his fog of confusion subsided, his voice became stronger, and his mood got better.

Dr. Dad is partially retired now and practices emergency medicine as his day job, so his guinea pigs are mainly himself, his family and friends. He is more enthusiastic than ever, though, about the field of medicine, and goes to conventions and conferences to learn more about wellness and bio-identical hormones.

So, who says an old dogtor can't learn new tricks?

NICE LEGS

Speaking of old dogs, have I mentioned that my husband is a native of St. Croix? Yah, mon. When we moved to Texas, he had to learn some Texas tricks, and this old dog didn't want to. It took a lot for him to find his inner Bubba-mon.

When we had lived in Texas less than two years, Eric and I celebrated our anniversary in Fredericksburg, a charming hamlet chock-a-full of German history in the Hill Country of Texas. Like anyone would, we planned our entire getaway around bicycling and running. However, given the fact that we'd just run the Texas marathon days before, it was very moderate bicycling and running.

Eric hadn't quite adjusted to Texas yet. Don't get me wrong. He liked Texas, but public outings with him scared me to death. Eric was always just a breath away from getting his ass whupped by a cowboy, because he is an incurable smartass.

Case in point: Eric and I met at work, and soon afterwards, he said to me, "Don't expect me to treat you like your shit doesn't stink just because everyone else here does." Charming. And then he asked me to marry him. I guess we know who won that round.

Where were we? Oh yes, driving through Llano, on the way to Fredericksburg. We were in the heart of Texas deer hunting country, and it just happened that we were smack in the middle of deer hunting season. As we drove into town, Eric put on his thickest, most sarcastic drawl and estimated the IQ and body weight of each ther-mal-camouflage-clad, beer-bellied hunter we passed. We pulled up to a gas pump, surrounded by converted SUVs and ATVs tricked out with gun turrets and swiveling Lazy Boys in their hacked-off back ends.

Eric put the car in park. "You're going to have to pump the gas."

Not to be a princess, but, "'Scuse me?" My husband never lets me lift a dainty little finger if he can help it. He'd have to be vomiting up a lung to ask me to pump gas.

He gestured at his bare legs and running attire. "I can't go out there like this."

"Because it's too cold?" I could understand this, seeing as it was January and all. That's why I had on full-length running tights. Duh.

"No, because . . ." He jerked his head toward the nearest hunter, garbed head-to-toe to withstand an arctic blast. "People will stare at me."

"Ahhhhhhh."

Eric's shorts were truly short; you know, the kind that shows 99.9% of your thighs? You see shorts like these on real runners in city parks. You do not see them in Llano, Texas. In Llano, real men don't wear sissy running shorts. Hell, real men don't run at all, in short shorts or anything else. Real men don't need to run, unless it's to the Allsup's for a six-pack of Lone Star beer. They get their exercise the manly way: they hunt and field-dress deer after they poke their dogies and till the back forty in their John Deeres. (My apologies to all aforesaid real men, 'cause I know there's a difference between a farmer and a cowboy, and never the twain shall meet.)

Well, I may have giggled and made a comment or two at this point, I dunno, but I did pump the gas. We passed more hunters on our way to a café where we planned to meet my mother for breakfast, like anyone would on their anniversary trip.

Um, yeah.

Anyway, Eric kept humming some dueling banjos song and talking about people who marry their first cousins. Then we pulled into the parking lot of the café.

Eric put the car in park. He turned a stricken face to me.

"Lotta hunters in there," I said before he had a chance to speak, gesturing towards the tiny, crowded restaurant and then at the giant vehicles around us. And I coughed to cover a chuckle.

"Har-de-har-har," said Eric.

"I think you're a little underdressed," I said, and this time I burst out laughing. Every person in the restaurant except my mom, who by now was waving cheerily at us through the window, was wearing thermal camo overalls.

We hurried into the bacon-scented café, Eric tugging in vain at his shorts. They were as long as they were going to get. All eyes followed us to the table, where Mom kissed and hugged us with noisy gusto.

As soon as we sat down, she asked Eric to run to her car and get something. Well, a man doesn't ever say no to his mother-in-law, does he? Eric took a deep breath and re-trod his walk of shame to the parking lot, wishing, I'm sure, for Harry Potter's invisibility cloak.

When he was out of earshot, I leaned in and whispered, "Mom, Eric is mortified about his running shorts."

"Why?" she asked. "He looks fine."

"Look around, Mom. Hunters. No short running shorts." I giggled. "He feels conspicuous."

My mother never wastes an opportunity, and the woman is quick. She turned to the nearest hunter, a healthy fellow of 270 pounds or so, 8.6 pounds of it in facial hair.

"Would you do me a favor?" she asked him.

Have I mentioned that my mother is a great source of genetic material? She is charming and pretty, and all men love her. This hunter was no exception.

"Why sure, ma'am, what can I do ya for?" he said, and damn if his voice wasn't a dead ringer for Eric's imitation hunter-drawl earlier.

"See that man in the running shorts out there in the parking lot? That's my son-in-law. He is a little embarrassed about wearing shorts. I was wondering if you could let out a big wolf whistle when he comes back in?"

He turned to his cronies, who were hanging on every word of this interchange. He brayed a laugh, and after a split second, so did his two friends. "I'd be delighted to help ya out, ma'am."

"Thank you sooooo much," she said, and turned back to her menu, a Mona Lisa smile on her face.

The front door opened, sounding its bell. My clean-shaven husband with his mighty fine exposed gams stepped in.

Without hesitating as long as it would take to load his 30.06 deer rifle, the hunter yelled out, "Hey boy, NICE LEGS!"

Eric looked around slowly, hoping the hunter was talking to someone else. His face lost all color. The restaurant grew so quiet you could almost hear the steam hissing out of Eric's ears. After a few beats, the café exploded in sound, as the hunter and his buddies cackled and whooped with laughter. They pounded the table, and one of them clapped our hunter on the back with a resounding thwump.

Eric tilted his head just enough to be perceptible and made the four quick strides from the door to our table, his naked legs eye-level as he pushed between two tables on the way. The hunter reached out and clasped his meaty paw around Eric's arm.

He hooked his thumb at my mother. "Yore mother-in-law put me up to it. I don't normally comment on another feller's legs."

"They are awful nice, though," one of his friends said, and they all set to hee-hawing again.

It is possible that Eric now finds this story humorous. At the time, he may or may not have planned the slow and painful death of his mother-in-law in the near future, although you'd never have known it then. Let's just say that when we drew up our house plans for our someday house on our property in Nowheresville, he didn't include a mother-in-law suite.

But he did let me buy him a pair of longer running shorts.

SURFSIDE EXPECTATIONS

Eric and I had our eye on the Texas Triple, three marathons that began with our already-completed New Year's Day Texas Marathon. Number two was the Valentine's Day Surfside Beach marathon. Unfortunately, we had to skip it when Eric got a hard poke in the eye and his doctor kiboshed running until a few days after the race, for fear that it would jar and tear his retina. Ouchie. We were tremendously depressed (race t-shirt! entrance fee! Texas Triple!), but we talked to the race organizer, who let us run it solo one week later, after the doctor had given Eric the go-ahead.

And so, on a cold and windy day in late February, we put another notch in our belts. The race was a 13.1-mile out-and-back run entirely on the flat, packed beach sand. Wicked awesome. We drove the course before dawn, stashing water bottles just out of the surf every couple of miles, getting as far as we could get from the smelly dead porpoise at mile six.

Unfortunately, some yay-hoo ran over and busted all our water bottles, so it was a very thirsty day. In your face, jerkwad: we finished anyway, and even got our t-shirts. Two down, one to go for the Texas Triple—triumph!

NO MOJO

I finished February strong, but by March, I was out of mojo. The combined effects of a lot of training on my forty-two-year-old body, which had only been doing endurance events for a year, plus the full-frontal assault of hormones and anxiety, were taking a heavy toll on me. I wasn't sure I'd be able to do the Seabrook Lucky Trails marathon, the third of the Texas Triple that I wanted so badly to finish. Dr. Dad told me to put away the training calendar until I was healed, but this went against everything in my psyche. When the going gets tough, the tough get going, right? Only the fittest survive.

But I was being told to walk, not run, to smell the roses, to spin, to glide, to sleep, and to listen to my body. When I huff and puff and fight my racing heartbeat during a walk, much less a two-mile run, then I am supposed to glean that something is wrong, that I should slow down. When I am dizzy, wobbly, and weak, I am to deduce that I am redlining my hormonal and physical reserves. Refortify the adrenal, rebuild the glycogen reserves, rest the thyroid, replenish the testosterone.

It sucked.

Not being able to train and race was impacting not just my own heart and mind, but my husband's, who wouldn't do it without me. And he needed exercise, not just races. Runs were emotional salve to him. In fact, on the occasion of our first date, he called me one hour beforehand and asked to push it back by an hour so he could go run. I thought, *Well, I guess that should tell me something.* It turned out that it said a lot. He was so scared about getting his words to me just right, that only a run could calm his nerves and center his brain. In the end, he did great: "You stop my heart," he said. It stopped mine. And I returned the favor for a guy like that by costing him his training and his races now? I felt like a troll.

I decided to lower my expectations. I'd still get credit for the marathon if I finished in eight hours, so if I had to, I determined to chuck my pride and jog/walk/walk/walk/jog/walk. Our Texas Triple t-shirts were riding on it.

TEXAS TRIPLE: BEEN THERE, DONE THAT

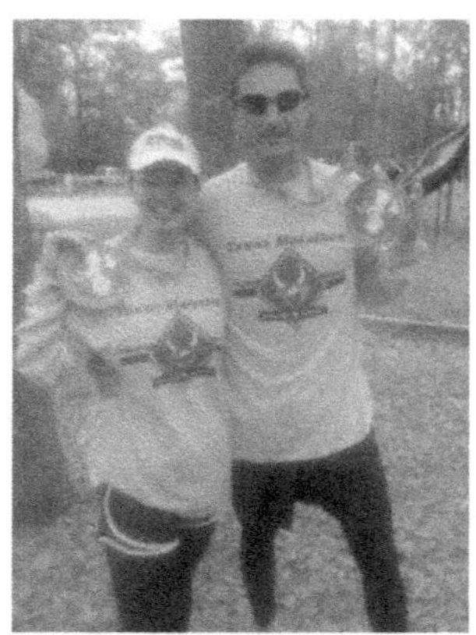

Above: Texas Triple Race #1: Texas Marathon on New Year's Day

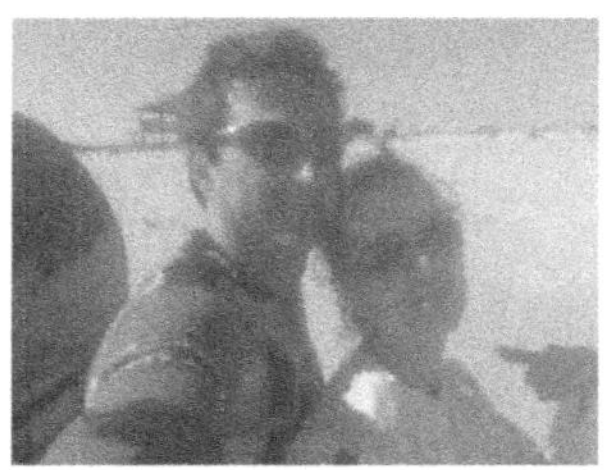

Above: Texas Triple Race #2 Surfside Marathon, solo, on a lovely February day

We had conquered the Texas Marathon on New Year's Day. We had rescheduled our Surfside Marathon from Valentine's Day to later in February, and salvaged our run at the Texas Triple by completing it without endangering Eric's eye. I had curtailed my training so that we had a chance to overcome my body breakdown and finish the mid-March Seabrook Lucky Trails Marathon, which would complete the Triple.

We formulated a plan, or rather I did, and Eric nodded in all the right places. Eric and I would start an hour and a half early with the other walkers, and even though it was not how we'd wanted it to end, we would walk the event.

It was pitch dark when we lined up to start the race. The weather was humid, which wasn't surprising on the Gulf Coast. Seabrook was a dirt trail course that ran along the sea line. The race trail was similar to the Texas Marathon—we would do four laps of a looped course. The trail ran partially along a bayou, and at one point, it crossed a swampy inlet on a bouncy wooden bridge. The turnaround was on the beach. We had trained on this course several times, and we loved it.

The walking start was pretty anticlimactic compared to other race starts. Usually, a gun goes off and hundreds or thousands of nervous racers shoot forward, all bunched together and feeding off each other's adrenaline, over-racing for the first several miles. For the walking start, we simply stood in a small pack in the dark until the organizer said, "Ready, set, go," and began walking with us.

The walk was lovely, for all of about three and a half minutes. Then I started to trot.

"What are you doing?" Eric asked as he slipped into a trot beside me.

"This is bullshit," I said.

"Pamela, don't overdo it. We have twenty-six miles to go," he said.

"Yeah, and we'll never get there at this pace. I feel fine. I promise I'll stop if I feel bad."

Luckily, it was dark, so I couldn't see Eric's expression. Another walker or two sped up to fall in with us. For forty-five minutes before dawn, we ran the soft dirt trails in complete silence. It was fantastic. We continued our small group lovefest and were well into our second loop before the mass of runners started. The fastest runners caught up with us immediately, but that was all right.

A week before, I couldn't run around the block. But on that day I ran twenty-six miles. Sure, we still walked a few sections at around miles twenty and twenty-four. Hey, so did the guy who won the race. In fact, I saw him vomiting, which I didn't do because I was not about to work that hard. Anyway, a few short walks didn't change the fact that this race was amazing, it was joyful, it was transcendent, it was a victory over my broken-down old body. Our time was halfway decent, too. It looked especially good since we crossed the finish line hand-in-hand, having started an hour and a half before the race clock did, which made it look like we were three-hours-and-change speed demons. Let's keep our true time a secret between you and us, OK?

The best part was yet to come. When we finished, we went to collect our Texas Triple prize. I expected a t-shirt. Au contraire. The award was a lined windbreaker with the Texas Triple logo and year embroidered on it. Serious bling! It's still my most prized garment.

We didn't have a great desire to marathon all the time—well, Eric did not have a great desire to marathon all the time—but we wanted to do more trail running and adventure racing. OK, that was still pretty much just me; Eric wanted to Ironman. I was intrigued by the ultramarathons, but one has to balance training time against the rest of life's commitments.

I kinda felt like a badass. At least for that moment. Next up: Half Ironman in April.

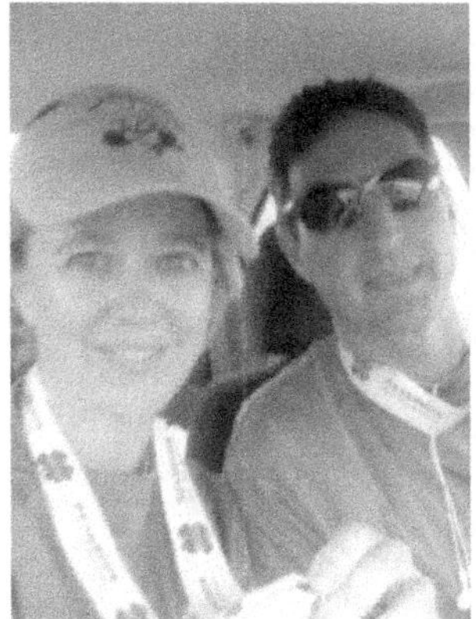

Above: Texas Triple Race #3 Seabrook in mid-March

BRING IT, PART DEUX

What started as a fascination with ultramarathons quickly morphed into a near obsession for me. Especially after we pulled another $300/no-t-shirt scratch on our April triathlon, due to my lingering post-Triple exhaustion. I had spent what little energy I had left on running Seabrook, and it took me six weeks before I had sufficient reserves to resume any kind of training again. I tried to talk Eric into just going out and doing the April Half Ironman on guts alone, like I'd done Seabrook, but he put his foot down. He was probably right, but by then, I was coming out of my skin with the need to train for something big. It wasn't long before I found us a . . . wait for it . . . ULTRAMARATHON TRAINING PLAN {http://run100miles.com/ultra-resources/50-mile-training-program/}!

At this point in our running careers, about one month after we completed the Texas Triple, we had run one 50K in addition to our three marathons; not a 50K race, but a 50K "Pamela and Eric training run" at Brazos Bend. By my stellar deduction, this meant that our next hurdle was the 50-miler. And, yes, by "our," I mean mine, because Eric was not enthusiastic about doing an ultramarathon. He went along with it, but only because I promised him trail running, also known as fast hiking, instead of road running. And who doesn't love hiking?

Our ultra plan called for two rest days, one short run day, three medium runs, and one long run each week. Does that add up to seven days? I hope so, but I got kind of lost for a moment. It spanned seventeen weeks. We set our sights on a February 50-miler at Huntsville State Park: the Rocky Raccoon. {We had accidentally competed in part of this race during November of the previous year. The organizers had moved it to February and increased the distance.} We would start the training program in October, from 50K readiness, which we would maintain over the summer and early fall.

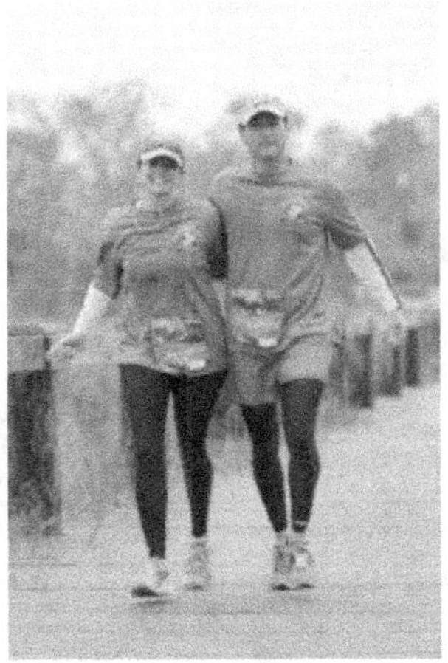

From everything I'd read about ultras, hydration, fuel, and walking are as important as running. We would follow the website's recommendation to walk ten out of every sixty minutes. Food, drink, and the call of nature fit into the walk segment. Every week would soon have four runs that were over an hour long, so we started working on our base fitness immediately.

Dr. Dad offered his input when I went over the plan with him: "You're going to cripple yourself, Pamela." But, really, what did he know, anyway?

Eric and I had to train together, which meant our teenagers would be on the lam in our absence. But our eldest at home had a driver's license by then, and my ex-husband lived in town, so we figured it was doable. If it weren't, it wouldn't be for lack of trying.

FASHION SHMASHION

There was a day, there was a time, when I cared a whole lot more about how I looked. I spent time and money on my hair, I wore makeup, and I selected my outfit each day from an overloaded closet organized by season, type of clothing, and color. And I looked good. Darn good. Because that's the woman my mother raised me to be.

At the age of almost forty-two, I was in the best shape of my life. I could wear the clothes I did as a teenager. I guess you could say I was aging pretty well, from outward appearances; not so well internally with the hormones, but hey, it's all about the outside, right?

Somehow, though, a very large collection of bicycle, triathlon, and marathon shirts and a rainbow selection of leggings had replaced my designer wardrobe. My mom was horrified.

Worse, I'd started cutting and coloring my own hair to save time . . . and then I'd wear it for days on end in Eric's favorite look: a scrunchy with the bangs twisted back into a miniature butterfly clip. But if you're working out twice a day, this makes sense, right? I am told that I used to pour baby powder on my hair as a teenager if I didn't have enough time to wash it. This memory brings tears of humiliation to my mother's eyes. I, however, recall nothing of the sort. Great idea, though.

I had used the same blush and powder for four years. Yes, you read that right. Not the same brands—the same exact containers. They looked like they'd last me a few more, too.

My beautiful jewelry was tucked neatly into its organizer, primarily because the only things I wore were the earrings my husband had bought me the previous summer. And my wedding ring. I thought my Texas Marathon giant bling medallion would look nice with my outfits, but it's a little heavy for everyday wear.

I dressed professionally for work when I had to—and thank the Lord that most of my work was done from home in my jammies on my laptop—but I whined about the hose and shoes. I'd lived in the Virgin Islands for six years; hose was practically illegal there.

Yes, gone was the nineteen-year-old me who would storm into the shower to wash and style my hair every time I entered my home. In its place was a woman who might look more disheveled, but was happier and healthier than she had ever been in her life.

Definitely a trade in my favor.

ROCKIN' 'N' ROLLIN'

"So, I'm thinking we should all sign up for the San Antonio Rock 'n' Roll Marathon and do it together," our daughter Marie said, apropos of nothing, the portrait of nonchalance.

We were sitting around watching ESPN together on a hot summer day at my parents' house. Eric and I had been telling her the story that morning about completing our third marathon in three months and earning our prized Texas Triple windbreakers. And I may have droned on about ultramarathons and trail running for an hour without a breath. OK, but *otherwise* apropos of nothing.

Marie had never completed a marathon—or a half marathon or any other running race—but she was a recently retired world-class swimmer. She'd swum endurance events from her early teens, and had once trained partway for a Half Ironman. She ran regularly, but not distance.

Marathons are not the activity of choice for most twenty-one-year-old girls. Even though I ran distance from the age of fifteen, I partied too hard at her age to run marathons. Not Marie. Marie was our serious child. She'd founded a non-profit when she was seventeen years old to help in the fight for better education for the youth of the Caribbean. She was now a junior in the prestigious Honors Humanities program at the University of Texas. Maybe a marathon wasn't such a big surprise for a girl like her.

"Wow, sure, yes," Eric and I stuttered.

Within minutes, I had signed us all up online and was handing out training programs. Marie would train in Austin, we would train in Houston, and never the twain should meet until San Antonio in November.

Eric and I were scheduled to do our trail ultra the next February, and we decided the Rock 'n' Roll marathon would fold nicely into our training schedule, so we changed our game. We moved our runs from asphalt to dirt, crushed rock, caliche, and gravel, to mud, sand, and grass . . . and unfortunately, to hummocks, hillocks, dips, depressions, bumps, stumps, stones, and holes.

Our Sunday long runs over the summer topped fifteen miles and kept getting longer, and years of floppy ankles caught up with me. I torqued and twisted them, especially the right one, over and over. Scorching white-hot pain plagued my instep, then migrated. My instep still hurt, but soon the base of my foot hurt, too, radiating back to what felt like a railroad spike through my heel.

My father didn't raise no sissy. Mind over matter. More Aleve. I kept going through the long, hot summer and into the fall. We didn't schedule any races, we just trained. Painfully, painfully trained. The month leading up to the Rock 'n' Roll really beat us up. Eric spent all of October in Canada for work, and his hours and six-day work weeks made training tough. Then he sprained his ankle, which didn't help, and the weather turned wintery and he got sick. Marie reported that her training was spotty, but she still felt she could do it. I trained alone back in Houston, and we hid our troubles from her. No reason to raise concerns.

The week before the Rock 'n' Roll, I did a solo marathon on a five-hour training pace on concrete along Buffalo Bayou in Houston, and the pain in my right foot was nearly unendurable. I stopped every six miles and texted Eric a photo. One thousand miles away, he ran his marathon in a state park near the Bay of Fundy, snapping pictures and texting them to me. We finished together, and he flew home the next day.

Between his coughs on our drive home from the airport, we compared notes.

"I don't think you should do this race, Pamela. I think you need to go to the doctor and figure out what's wrong with your foot," Eric said.

"You're one to talk, sick boy with the sprained ankle," I retorted.

"I have no business doing this marathon," he said.

"Nor do I," I said.

"So are you gonna scratch?" he asked.

"Are you out of your mind? My college-age stepdaughter asked me to do a marathon with you guys. I would run across nails to do this."

Eric smiled. "Yeah, same here."

And so the next week, we lined up at the start with a sweetly nervous Marie, and off we went. It was my worst marathon finish ever: five hours and forty minutes was forty minutes slower than my training run a week before, and a race should be at least ten percent faster than a training run. Plus I had an ugly mood swing as the pain rocked me, and I lashed out at everything around me, including Eric, who got in trouble with me for nothing more than expressing his support imperfectly. After I caught back up with him (because he left my ass when I was bitchy), Eric held my hand when the waves came over me, mostly to keep me from swinging at anyone. It made an impact on some spectators, though. We saw the same people several times during the course, and they always yelled, "Look, it's the couple that holds hands while they run." Ha! If they only knew.

I know it sounds like it was awful, but I will tell you the truth: It was wonderful. It was a top-rung parenting and athletic experience. I wouldn't trade my fastest runs on my fittest days in the best of conditions for that death march with Marie.

It was hard for all of us, though, not just me. Marie learned about the twenty-mile wall, where even twenty-one-year-old women suddenly don't believe there is any way they can put one foot in front of the other enough times to finish six more miles.

"You can do it, Marie," Eric urged her. "Just keep walking, and any time you feel like you may live, run. It happens to everyone at twenty miles, every race. Some people just look faster getting through it."

"We call it the death shuffle," I added. "Use as little energy as you can and shuffle along. Forward motion. It will be over soon."

Along with us, Marie experienced the humiliation of seeing an old, limping fat woman pass her. Of the rock-n-roll bands finishing their set and packing up before you reached them on the back of the course. She discovered that training counts, but heart matters more.

We suffered together in the unseasonable heat and humidity, but we finished—almost together. In a streak of expected competitive spirit, Marie passed us one minute before the finish line. Gotta love that in her. She was glowing.

I would endure the pain in San Antonio a thousand times again for the thrill and satisfaction of completing that race with my husband and stepdaughter. Top ten stepmom moment, for sure.

IDENTITY THEFT

And so it was that over the last six months leading up to the marathon with Marie that plantar fasciitis had snuck into my life. Now, it tried to steal my identity. I'm a mediocre, middle-aged triathlete, and I am a runner. In the space of the past year, I had run five marathons and trained for a trail ultra. I'd come a long way, and I was proud of myself—and then it was over.

Despite my iron will and a rigorous training schedule, I was still subject to the reality of my body. I am hyperflexible and have hyper-mobile joints, weak hips, and weak ankles. When I started flopping along on uneven trails for sixty miles every week, my chronic and annoying foot pain became almost crippling. My doctor told me to give it a rest.

Overnight I went from running sixty miles a week to sitting still. The withdrawal from runner's high hurt and left me even more emotionally erratic than usual, and the weight gain frustrated me (the hell you say I can't have bread pudding with chocolate sauce after every meal anymore!). My orthopedist's condescending advice infuriated me: "Be patient, don't run, I'll see you in a year. Try thera-pies if you want, but nothing will work. It's not like you're a real athlete anyway."

OK, he didn't say those exact words, but they were close.

My diagnosis crushed Eric. To him, exercising is not the same as racing. He won't call himself a triathlete unless he *competes*. He won't compete if he doesn't run. And he won't run or race without me, which made him sort of sad and crazy, like me. A double whammy.

I was able to bike, and I was encouraged to swim. I hate to swim; and who wants to wear a bathing suit when they've gained weight? So it looked like there would be a lot of bicycling in my near future. This actually worked for Eric. He loved bicycling so much that ten years ago he opened a bike shop. Which became a triathlon shop. Which turned into a chain of GNCs with attached bicycle/triathlon shops. Which lost a ton of money and kept him from bicycling for a few years. If that isn't love, I don't know what is.

I not only couldn't run, but even walking was difficult. We went to the Houston Livestock Show and Rodeo and a Kenny Chesney concert, and just walking from the car to the stadium and through the fairgrounds caused gasp-out-loud throbbing pain. That's about lifestyle and identity though, not about functionality. I'm aware that I am blessed compared to others with worse injuries and conditions. This did not stop me from whining about it, of course. Especially because—and isn't this ironic?—my hormones weren't all that awful at that time. Argh!

I wanted to run again. I wanted to ultramarathon; I wanted to Ironman. So, I couldn't just do nothing and pray for a recovery. Whether my ortho thought it worked or not, I had to do physical therapy (ultrasound, massage, ART, hot tub, and ice) with Dr. Death at the House of Pain. Trust me, that was worse than natural child-birth. They must do something right there, though, because half the Houston Rockets were in the waiting room with me at any given visit. And, yes, Yao Ming really is that tall.

I had quite a thrapy routine on my own, too: Strassberg sock at night, stretching, ankle strengthening, Aleve, orthotics, special shoes —I did it all. Patiently (for me).

Long term, I knew I should give up our beloved but uneven trails in favor of flatter terrain. I could still run with the gators at Brazos Bend someday, but only on the groomed trails. And I needed to forget about the ultras. Even more, I needed to re-engineer my running style and switch to minimalist shoes, as it was now clear that my highly-structured wedge-style running shoes were largely to blame for my condition. (Well, that and overtraining on uneven terrain, but I'd rather blame the shoes.) They caused me to run with a heel strike. I needed to switch to shoes that moved my weight forward to the front or middle of my foot.

And so I pledged no more identity theft, and I began micro-runs in Vibram's Five Fingers, the little "glove" shoes. I had to visualize and adopt a new form; I had to retrain my body. "Weight forward, no heel strike, weight forward, no heel strike, weight forward, no heel strike," I chanted as I plodded along in my new VFFs.

Happy trails to all you runners out there. I'm jealous. But I'm on my way back.

IF I CAN BEAT THIS, I CAN BEAT PLANTAR FASCIITIS.

I made a decision a few years ago that changed my life for the better, forever: I drank alone for the last time. I drank *too much*, alone, and damaged my relationships and myself for the last time.

My eight-year-old son, Clark Kent the ADHD WonderKid, had told his teacher that he was worried about his mother. When his teacher called me in for a conference, I was stopped cold. Clark was right. I had been drinking too many Bloody Marys too often for too many years. My face was puffy, I woke up hungover too many times to count, and still, I cut out of work early to drink wine with my girl-friends. I was an awful drunk, and I didn't have the bandwidth to deal with my kids' issues. And of course, I wasn't exercising, but I didn't care enough about me to do anything about it. I tried cutting back any number of times, for all the good it did. But I would do almost anything for my kids.

So I told my boss I would see him in ten days. He didn't ask why, which said a lot. I boarded a plane for St. Lucia and I checked into a mind and body spa for a week of rejuvenation while I dried out. I'm not a joiner; I wish I was, but I'm not. AA was not for me. So, St. Lucia, solo.

So what did I do when I got there?

Got drunk in my room on everything in the minibar, in a

panicked, sobbing frenzy. So drunk that I woke up the next morning and didn't remember falling asleep in the bathtub with the TV on. I didn't think I could get lower than I had been after I heard Clark's words from his teacher, but that did it.

The morning after the last time I drank alcohol was the lowest point of my life. It beat out my later divorce, the bloody aftermath, and the custody battle that ensued. I despised myself, and not for the first time, I wished I were selfish enough to kill myself. It seemed like that would be so much easier.

For me. But this was not about me. It was about my kids.

So, I picked myself up and put on my too-tight stretchy exercise clothes that used to fit and marched with gritted teeth up seven thousand steps in the heat to the mind and body center. I spent the remaining six days (instead of the planned seven) alone in my mind. My version of Elizabeth Gilbert's year of eating, praying, and loving, I guess. I sweated. I cried. I replayed Clark's words and my failures over and over in my mind. I felt like absolute crap. I walked the beaches until my feet were as smooth as a baby's bottom. And then I came home dry.

It was hard. So very, very hard.

My husband drank quite a lot at the time, and he didn't slow down for me. The bad marriage I had drowned in booze was impossible to tolerate without anesthetic and contributed to my urge to drink. Most of my friends were heavy drinkers, too, and they viewed my decision to stop drinking as a personal indictment of their choices.

Who was this about, anyway? Right. My kids. I kept going.

I counted the days out painfully, one by one. I again rejected the idea of AA, not only because of my anti-joiner bent, but out of fear of the impact it would have on my high-profile career in our small community. I did it alone, with only one real friend who was aware and still with me *(thanks, Nat!)*, in the middle of the Cruzan Rum-rich island environment of St. Croix, USVI.

Years later, three months had passed. Alcohol abstinence started getting easier—not a lot easier, but easier. And I felt better, I looked better. I lost weight. I acted nicer. I became more energetic and productive, crisper. I started running again, and Clark quit worrying about me.

I am now married to a man who gave up alcohol on our first date. The same date on which he told me I stopped his heart. Eric wasted (pardon the pun) no time in showing me he meant to be my hero, and he is, for more by far than putting up with me writing about his Ironman underwear.

People ask me how I do it all. I don't know. But I do know that a drunken Pamela could not have run five marathons and written two novels in one year while parenting and holding down a day job, even with the world's greatest husband.

I'd love to say that after this many years dry that I never think about drinking, but that is not true. Sometimes I wake up with the sweats, dreaming that I have fallen off the wagon. In those dark moments in the middle of the night, I long to search the house for a bottle of comfort. Every time I travel, the urge strikes, because I used to drink alone in hotel rooms. Now, instead, I sit awake all night, writing to distract myself and praying for the day I never travel alone again.

I don't want to waste another day or night of my life. I want to be the best me I can be 24/7, for my kids, my husband, and finally, for myself—so I can meet my goals, important and physically challenging goals like endurance triathlons and marathons. I know only one way to do this, so I will stay true. One day at a time. One year at a time. For the rest of my life.

MY DIET IS NOT A RACIST.

I am a lifestyle follower of the "no white" diet, but it's not a racist and neither am I. Big difference. Get it straight, people!

Also, I have heard whispering behind my back that I should practice what I preach or not throw stones in a glass house or some other cliché-ridden B.S., and I have just one thing to say about THAT, y'all, as a writer and a human being: I totally know! I am the embodiment of the word "binge." Can you say Cinnabon? But, I swear, I repent and shall stray only occasionally more.

So, what I do, and have done for years—years at a time, even—is eat no white foods. It's kinda like the Pamela version of Paleo, although I've read far too little about Paleo and am mostly going by what other people tell me, which I've heard is a bad idea, but whatever. Note: I am not a doctor, but my doctor recommended I follow a Paleo lifestyle. My way is not the way for all. It just works for me. So here goes nothing:

The Chunky Phase: "Ass the Size of Delaware"—2 weeks

No sugar, no flour, no rice, no potatoes, no pasta, no fruit. I also avoid simple-carb veggies (the sweetest-tasting ones) like corn, carrots, and sweet peas. Don't cheat! If you do, you'll gain weight, not lose it. Avocado and exotic oils like hazelnut, brazil nut, avocado (the oil in addition to the fruit) are a yes on this diet, as is ghee (butter from grass-fed cows with the casein and lactose removed), nuts in moderation—good fats are fine, bad fats are always bad fats. The leaner the meat, the better, but all meat (and eggs) will work on this diet. I try to go by the three-ounce portion size rule for proteins. A vegetable serving size is one cup, but leafy greens are two cups. I visualize my plate, and of the food on it, 1/3 is protein (into which I group nuts, eggs, and meat, in my simple mind) and 2/3 are veggies, with the protein about the size and thickness of my hand.

I avoid lentils and beans in this phase—they're good carbs, but still too carby for breaking the hold bad carbs have on me. The first four days, have Excedrin handy because you will have bitchin' headaches along with your carb cravings as you go into withdrawal. But after four days, you will not be hungry. Drink tons of water.

Oh, a bonus: you're eating unprocessed food that is gluten-free, and eliminating yucky yeast in your digestive system, which can farg your health up in about a million ways. Read more about yeast and you at the Hotze Health & Wellness Center's website {http://www. hotzehwc.com}, from the geniuses and saints who saved me from myself with bioidentical hormones. If you go whole hog and buy grass-fed, hormone- and antibiotic-free, and free-range on your meats/eggs, and organic on your veggies, you're talking health explosion. Try it. Your body will thank you.

General success tips below. *If you do this right, ladies will lose eight to twelve pounds, and men, ten to fifteen pounds. And you're losing fat, not water.*

The Less-Chunky Phase: "I can open my eyes halfway when I'm naked"—2 weeks (or however long it takes)

No sugar, no flour, no rice, no potatoes, no pasta. I sparingly add back in all fruits and veggies except bananas, which are the fruits most easily converted to sugar. The best fruits on this type of diet? Those with seeds: strawberries, kiwis, raspberries, blackberries. I also throw in beans and lentils in this phase, in moderation. They're a good carb! You're still low-yeast, unprocessed, and gluten-free in this phase, and hopefully chemical-, antibiotic-, and hormone-free as well. Now the food on my plate is 1/3 protein, 2/3 fruit and vegetables, but going heavy on the vegetables.

The Lifestyle Phase: "Damn, I think I look pretty good"—forever, or until you succumb to a giant apple fritter at Friday's Fried Chicken Restaurant in Shiner, Texas

No sugar, no flour, but add back in brown rice, SWEET potatoes, quinoa, even some corn-based pasta occasionally. Those following Paleo as a religion just screamed, "NO!!!" But I told you, this is Pamela Paleo. Eat this way forever. *It's good for you.* Also, if you are careful, you can stay gluten-, hormone-, antibiotic-, and chemical-free in this stage, too. Watch for processed foods (like pasta) and pick the natural alternatives, or just don't eat processed at all. In this phase, your yeast count has gone up, but it's at a minimal, probably acceptable level.

How does your plate look now? You are still basically 1/3 protein an 2/3 fruit and veggies, but over the day I'll have the equivalent of 1 portion of starches. If I'm working out like a fiend, I'll increase the starches as needed, basically until I feel my energy level is sufficient to sustain me through rigorous and lengthy training sessions.

General advice for not swelling up like a hippopotamus

If you must use sweeteners, minimize them. They are ASS SWELLERS. And NEVER USE chemical sweeteners. I have suffered intense joint pain using sucralose. Aspartame kills lab rats and gives me horrid headaches. The last thing I want is dead rats on my conscience when I have a migraine. Fruit purees, honey, agave, coconut, and maple syrup/sugar work well—hint, hint. If you're having trouble losing weight, you can substitute in xylitol (natural, low-calorie sweetener) or pure, real stevia from the leaf. I recently learned the hard way that due to the stevia craze, unscrupulous manufacturers are processing the stevia and cutting it with a chemical. Yeah. Before I discovered this, it also gave me joint pain from swelling. Don't believe me? Google it. You'll find growing reports from real humans about this phenomenon.

Can't live without breading on your meat? If you must fry, and fry with breading, try substituting ground nuts or almond flour for regular flour. I like ground sesame seeds, too, although cleaning the food processor keeps me from doing it very often. Bob's Red Mill has great almond flour and garbanzo (chickpea) flour. I use their quinoa flour for pancakes and for cupcakes. I use garbanzo for savory dishes. You could even go crazy and fry in coconut oil or, for a really high temperature alternative to olive oils, ghee. Second best: exotic oils. And the old guy (Bob) that owns Bob's Red Mill gave his company to his employees, which is so cool I can't stand it.

Need speedy snacks that don't spoil? Try the delicious Larabars or the Epic line of meat bars. Don't mock the meat bars. If you like beef jerky, you'll love them. Plus you'll feel like a Native American eating pemmican, which works for me since I was o-b-s-e-s-s-e-d with Indians as a child.

Hydrate, hydrate, hydrate. Water, tea, or fruit-sweetened drinks. Coffee and tea. Go crazy with your tea and try something new, like fennel or ginger tea, which are two of my faves. We also drink a lot of coconut water (post workout) and cold-pressed apple juice, which I dilute with water until there's just a hint of favor. Speaking of Hint, they make a great line of unsweetened flavored waters, as does Metromint. You can duplicate these at home in a pitcher by adding herbs, cacao, fruit, and veggies.

Cutting sugar means cutting it from everything. Check your cough drops and cold meds—big time sugar. I switched to caplets instead of my beloved hot Theraflu when I did this. And there are also naturally sweetened cough drops to help you stay away from artificially sweetened ones.

Watch for hidden sugars, artificial sweeteners, chemicals, and processing. If you can't pronounce it, that's a bad sign. Learn to read labels for a product's total carb count. Red pasta sauce in the grocery store has a lot of sugar (and processed-y preservative-y stuff), as do ketchup and peanut butter. Look for natural, low-carb alternatives, make your own, or do without. Better yet, go for almond, cashew, pecan, walnut, or (orgasmically delicious) macadamia nut butter. Even sunflower tastes pretty good. My top choice: Kolat nut butters, mixed with yummy stuff like blueberries, cinnamon, vanilla, chocolate, coconut, and espresso. My favorite is their almond butters. Salad dressings contain a lot of filler, and low fat usually means high sugar. Why not make your own? A little balsamic and dijon rocks. Lemon, oil, salt and pepper isn't bad either.

When you go to the grocery store, shop the outside aisles, away from the processed foods. You are returning to eating like a hunter-gatherer, to the way people used to eat before our society turned to white sugar and processed foods and got F-A-T. Think *whole* foods, all that good fibery stuff.

If your breath gets icky in the initial phases of Pamela Paleo, be careful of sugar and carbs in mouthwashes, gum, and mints. Read the labels and shop for alternatives. Xylitol-sweetened gums, mouthwashes, and even toothpastes are available online.

Stay off alcohol in the first two weeks, then when you add it back, go with the drinks with the least sugar or you'll really mess yourself up. Red wine and low-carb beer are good choices, but the less alcohol you drink, the more control you'll have over your weight, as alcohol is a simple-sugar-based liquid.

If you quit losing weight or start regaining it, pull out the simple carbs, which are the foods most easily converted to sugar.

As with any attempt to jumpstart your metabolism, eat smaller meals five or six times a day.

If you're an athlete, you may feel funny at first, but over time, your body will adjust. And, of course, you never take out carbs altogether, just worthless carbs. The more you exercise, the quicker you'll lose weight and be able to add the nutritious carbs back to your diet. I am a crappy middle-aged endurance athlete, and I can keep it really low-carb and still perform.

Supplements rock, no matter which diet you are on. My favorite multivitamin? Synergy. It's not only a comprehensive power pack with fantastic ingredients in a powdered capsule (think "easily metabolized") form, but it's also low-carb. Confession: I buy my vitamins pre-packaged for morning, noon, and night straight from the Hotze line. It's a little more expensive, but so easy.

Want to curb hunger with energy-sustaining, no-calorie protein? Try unflavored gelatin. I dissolve it in warm water, then I add flavor and ice cubes to the water.

Vinegars are secretly yeast breeders. Apple cider vinegar with the mother is okay in initial phases. Over time I add coconut vinegar, and occasionally some exotic ones like rice.

I swear by ascorbic acid (unbuffered vitamin C). Every morning, I add it to diluted cold- pressed apple juice, and sometimes I add fiber. Fiber is a good thing because it neutralizes carbs, and it also helps buffer the C. If you are not getting a lot of roughage, you should probably add in the fiber, or factor in an extra hour of bathroom time each day once you start this diet. If your stomach doesn't like the ascorbic acid, drink it with a meal with carbs, or cut down the amount. Same thing if you find yourself running to the bathroom a lot.

Love smoothies and other dishes that need added protein? You can find awesome pea, hemp, and beef proteins on Vitacost.

Last tip: if you suffer from adrenal fatigue or have a gripey stomach, I've adapted two concoctions from the *Trim Healthy Mama* book for these issues that are Pamela Paleo-friendly, and Eric drinks both every day. Here are the recipes:

Adrenal Enhancer

Adrenal support. Helps when you sleep too little, and stress and work too much.

2 lemons or 1 lemon and 1 grapefruit, peeled with pith left on

2- to 3 cups water (2 if grapefruit is used)

1 heaping teaspoon non irradiated turmeric powder

1 teaspoon ginger

2 to 3 tablespoons powdered alfalfa

1 tablespoon apple cider vinegar

1 tablespoon extra-virgin coconut oil (I use the dried version from Quest)

2 teaspoons protein powder

1/2 cup coconut cream

3 generous pinches of high-mineral salt like Celtic sea salt

2 tablespoons vanilla extract

1 teaspoon cinnamon

1/3 cup xylitol, honey, agave, maple syrup, maple sugar, or coconut sugar

Optional: 4 to 8 drops of therapeutic grade essential oil of lemon, 1 teaspoon fish oil

ADD:

8000 mg vitamin C (I use ascorbic acid)

Optional: 2 packets Unicity Balance (fiber, helps promote lower cholesterol and healthy weight and regularity; you can get it on Amazon. Eric's doctor has him on it—it replaced his Crestor prescription because of its red rice yeast component, and it worked)

Optional: 2 scoops N.O.-XPLODE pre-workout

Optional: 2 tablespoons liquid glucosamine/chondroitin if you want joint support

Blend citrus and water; strain. Put strained liquid back in blender and add other ingredients. Blend. Serve cold. Can be frozen for up to two weeks.

MAKES 2 DRINKS OF 30 OUNCES EACH

Gripey Gut Fixer
Enhances gut function, vitality, energy, and regularity.

3 cups water

3 bags oolong or green tea

3 tablespoons extra-virgin coconut oil (solid or powdered)

10 ounces plain, unsweetened kefir

1 scoop protein powder

1/2 cup cocoa

3 shakes vanilla extract

Generous pinch sea salt

1 teaspoon cinnamon

1 cup frozen fruit

1/3 cup xylitol, honey, agave, maple syrup, maple sugar, or coconut sugar

5 cups fresh greens (collard, turnip, spinach, kale, parsley, cilantro, anything!)

Optional: 1/8 cup powdered colostrum (We use Sovereign Labs, available on Amazon. Amazing for pet allergies, I use it at my doctor's request, and it has me able to hold cats, where before they gave me hives)

Boil water and tea bags vigorously and let sit, until warm.

Assemble ingredients. You need a Vitamix blender or a powerful smoothie machine for this.

Add 1 to 2 cups of tea and the EVCO (which emulsifies in the warm tea). Add the other ingredients. Blend for 2 minutes on a fairly high setting.

Add more tea or water to taste and sip all day long. Note: the woman that originated a recipe this is based on adds LOTS of water and makes it last all day. Eric doesn't. He drinks it with maybe ½ cup more liquid added.

My Sample Chunky-Phase Eating Plan
Breakfast:
Eggs with Rotel tomatoes. Chia pudding made with almond milk and vanilla.

Snack:
Frequent, tasty snacks are the only way I can stick with this diet, and luckily, there's a world of yummy options. Here are a few: 8 macadamia nuts, raw green veggies, a tablespoon of nut butter.

Note to those of you with very little brainpower (oh, sorry—*will power*): choose only one for each snack time.

Lunch:
Lettuce wraps with avocado, turkey, mayo & mustard, and raw veggies.

Snack:
Probably twice in the afternoon in the first four days; see snack ideas above.

Dinner:
A slab of meat (which gets smaller every day, but is large when I'm starving in the beginning) and cooked green veggies.

So that's it! My non-racist diet. I hope some of what works to keep me from flattening my own bicycle tires helps you, too.

DON'T STOP THE CARNIVAL, BICYCLING-STYLE.

Written by Eric, my personal coach, physical therapist, and nutritional consultant.

For six years, I was the co-owner of a small bike shop on St. Croix in the U.S. Virgin Islands. I was also the mechanic. And the custodian. And the nearly-everything-else. I did this and worked seventy hours a week at my day job. Sounds insane, and it felt like it, too. One store became multiple stores on multiple islands, adding to the insanity.

Very few people make money owning bike shops, and I sure didn't. I opened a shop because I had a passion for bikes and riding. I liked the people and the cycling culture. It's a fraternity that can include a hundred-and-twenty-pound Seattle racer with head-to-toe tattoos on a LiteSpeed and an old Rastaman who uses his Huffy to get his fruits to the market.

I soon learned, though, that running a bike shop had an unintended consequence: I worked while everyone else rode. In the ten years before opening the shops, I did about thirty triathlons. In the six years I owned the shops, I did zero.

Island bike shops are different from mainland bike shops. For island locals, the size of the bike meant the diameter of the wheel, never mind the frame. And bigger was always better. Size was directly linked to masculinity. Most Virgin Islands men were insulted if I tried to sell them a bike that fit, or from which they could dismount off the front of the seat without racking their privates and leaving their toes four inches off the ground. Heavier was better, too. The locals lived in constant fear that the aluminum or, heaven forbid, carbon-fiber frame would collapse under their weight and awesome power.

The roads on the islands were nearly all bad, so the idea of riding on a twenty-three-millimeter tire with a skinny rim was simply folly. You practically had to put the bikes on Fatboy tires to survive a ride without multiple flats.

Virgin Islanders speak an English dialect most people from the mainland can barely understand, peppered with a lot of island-specific terminology. When one of my first customers came in asking for a star, it took a while to figure out he wanted a gear from a rear cassette, and a while longer to re-establish my credibility.

Our shop sponsored local bicycle races and triathlons. When a good friend of mine showed up on the morning of his first triathlon, which included a one-mile ocean swim, his dreadlocks were stuffed into a swim cap that looked like a basketball glued to his head, and his entire body was covered in white zinc oxide paste. When I asked him about the zinc he laughed and said, "Eric, mon, everybody know dat black people dem can't swim."

St. Croix hosts an annual triathlon with qualifying slots for the Hawaii Ironman. In one of the early races, another West Indian who went by the singular name "Bongo" wore a full snorkel mask, large fins, and a life jacket for the ocean swim. The professional triathletes from all over the world, sleek in their Speedos and racing goggles, got quite a kick out of that.

Anyone who has traveled with bikes knows what airlines can do to them. The destruction is multiplied by ten when the destination is the Caribbean. I pulled a lot of all-nighters putting the pieces back together for overseas athletes before races. It took small miracles to make them roadworthy, and I often stole parts off my own bikes, only to have some off-island owners whine about how the bar tape was no longer pristine.

One year, a young, bushy-haired, soft-spoken pro named Michael Lovato {http://www.michaellovato.com} arrived twenty-four hours before the race with his rear derailleur broken in half, which jeopardized his hope of a top ten finish to generate some food money. I gave him the derailleur gratis off the best bike I had in the shop and sent him on his way with a box of PowerBars. He finished in the money. To this day, we exchange emails and remain friends. He has become a real force in the triathlon world, and I consider my contribution of a derailleur well spent.

The shops were unfortunately hit by the explosion of internet shopping and catalog houses like Performance and Colorado Cyclist. I'd be in the shop wrenching on a bike with the place full of customers when some yahoo would brag to everyone how he saved a hundred dollars buying his high-end road bike through the internet. And then, two months later, he would bring in his damaged shipping box containing a frame and two hundred parts that required actual tools and know-how to assemble. I charged him two hundred dollars to put it together. And with him standing there, I would cheerfully remind the customers that they got free tune-ups on any bikes purchased in the shop.

Many customers dragged in their mass-market K-Mart bikes to get the wheels straightened, the brakes to function, and the bike actually to shift gears. When they found out the work would cost more than they paid for the bike, I was the bad guy. "Waiiiiiiiit a minute," I would say. "I didn't sell you that piece of junk disguised as a bicycle in the first place."

I do believe there is a place for mass-market bicycles. If you have a kid that is growing like a weed and likely to hop off the bike in the front yard, let it crash into the bushes, and leave it there for weeks until she needs it again, there is no sense investing in a high-quality bike. But if you are buying a bike with the intention of riding it regularly, you can pay now or pay later.

The pleasure of owning those island bicycle shops is something I will pay for (literally) the rest of my life. I could be bitter over the money I lost, and sometimes I am, a little. However, it was gratifying to put over a thousand good bikes into small island communities. Before the shops, a typical local bike race would have four or five riders in it, including me. The concept of a peloton or a breakaway group had little meaning. During our final year, it was common to have sixty riders in three categories. That was pretty cool. Maybe not cool enough to justify the money lost, but still something I can hold onto with pride.

The most important concept I got from owning a bike shop in the islands was the importance of the local shop to the bicycling community. And it is thus with an appreciation for their value and their owners' sacrifice that I will forever support small bicycle shops. In the long run, I'll actually recoup the value of the money I invest in supporting those shops, unlike with my Caribbean stores.

Happy cycling, mon.

FREE YOUR MIND

Y ou never know where you will be when inspiration strikes. Driving down the freeway during rush hour? Trying to sleep in the middle of the night? Cooking dinner?

As a writer, I consciously place myself in the settings that are most likely to stimulate my creativity. Unfortunately for me, my creativity peaks when I exercise. When I bicycle, swim, or run, my tension eases. As my tension eases, my mind empties and makes room for new ideas to form. Before I consciously realize the process has even begun, it begins to refill itself.

Eric and I talked through the entire plot of my novel *Finding Harmony* one Saturday morning while out riding in Comanche County, Texas. The problem, though, is how to capture the ideas I get when I am bicycling at twenty-three miles per hour.

This dilemma used to be a roadblock to me, but not anymore. I got an iPhone with a voice memo app on it that allows me to voice-record and email the audio file to myself. Holy cow! I have my iPhone with me at all times, anyway. It fits in the bento bag on the frame of my bicycle. I can leave it in my swim bag on the side of the pool. I can run with it in my fuel belt. It's right at hand when I'm driving (no typing required).

Once, Eric and I were doing a four-hour ride at Brazos Bend State Park. As we pedaled along, we passed four deer on our right. There were yellow wildflowers on both sides of the road. On our left a seven-foot alligator sunned in the shallows of an algae-covered pond (I've circled him in the picture above). About halfway through this beautiful, mind-freeing ride, my brain bombarded me with ideas for improvements on my novel *Going for Kona*. I slowed down to talk them through with my husband. His questions generated more ideas.

I pulled out my iPhone. Three clicks later, without even pulling over, I had captured the good stuff without sacrificing date time with Eric or a great workout in a beautiful place. Whether it's book ideas or a grocery list, there's no need to sacrifice my ride time to sit at home with a pencil and paper. One more obstacle in the way of training removed.

DOUBLE DUTY

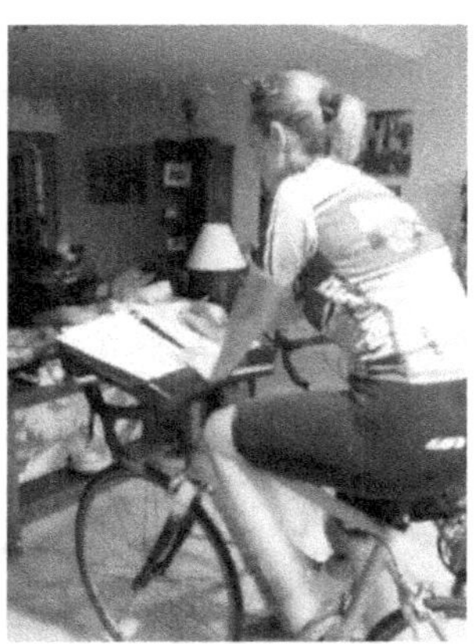

Editing must go on, as must my three-hour bike rides when I am preparing for the MS 150 ride from Houston to Austin. I need the time in my own saddle on my own bike, but one year during this training ramp-up I had to spend all weekend at the DFW Writers' Conference (yay!), so riding outside was not an option. Neither was frittering away three hours of editing time. My engineer husband rigged my lap desk to my aerobars with a bra strap to create the perfect ride-write space. Ingenuity!

My Ironman cousin Bud zip-ties a wireless mouse and keyboard to his lap desk while riding, with his laptop on a stool beside him. I added that to Eric's honey-do list.

BIKE TIPS FOR REAL PEOPLE

Bicycling is a learned sport that can overwhelm the novice. I had a live-in expert, thank goodness, who swooped in with answers and fixes whenever I had problems. Most of you aren't this lucky, so here's most of everything I learned from him:

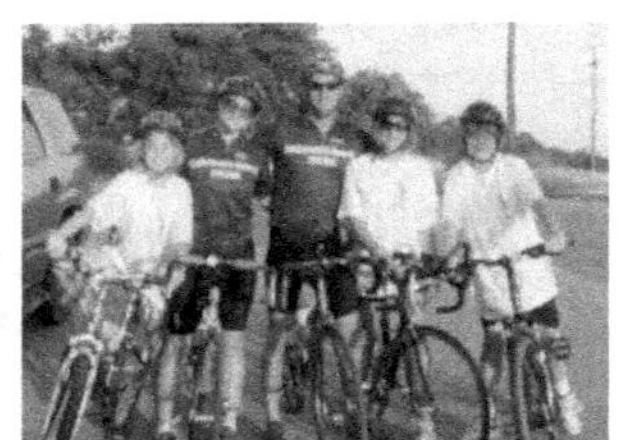

<u>BIKE TIP #1</u>

Bike fit is key. You will go faster and farther on a cheap bike that fits than a high-priced one that doesn't. This is where a good bike shop is so important. I am a huge advocate of finding expert help that you can trust in this area. This is not something you can just read up on, or trust your other novice bike friends to help you with. Some shops have incredibly sophisticated systems for fit, some use crusty old guys like me with a calibrated eyeball. Either way, take the time and do this right. Also, avoid this very common mistake: don't go to a [brand names interchangeable] Trek bike shop, get sized as a 56 cm, and then go on line and buy a 56 cm Fuji expecting them to be exactly the same. They are not.

*Warning, this next comment is based on Eric's personal opinion and may be subject to some debate from other experts.*I recommend that if you are borderline between sizes, you choose the smaller size. First of all, you can make a bike "bigger" by raising the seat, moving it back on its rails, changing the angle and length of the stem and the number of spacers under it. However, you can't make a bike much smaller. In addition, by simple logic, the smaller frame is lighter. The smaller frame will also be easier for you to handle on curvy roads.

Bike Tip #2

Don't underestimate the importance of seat height and cleat position on the shoe, when it comes to power transfer and prevention of injury. While this is related to fit, it can still be screwed up, even if you have the right-size bike. Go to a shop and get help.

In general, your pedal cleat should be under the ball of your foot, and positioned (left to right) such that your shoe is not rubbing on the crank arm as it rotates by. The angle of the cleat should be such that your feet are parallel with the bike—however, be careful. Everyone's anatomy is different, and it is possible that your natural, comfortable rotating position has your toes pointed either slightly in or slightly out. Getting this right is very important to reducing risk of injury. The main thing here is that as you rotate the pedals (do this in a training stand with no resistance so you can feel your legs move through the pedaling circle), you don't feel like your natural movement is being bound in one direction or the other. There is something called "float" used in the description of cleats and pedals. Float is a design feature that allows your heel to move left and right while your shoe is clipped into the pedal. More float means more freedom of lateral movement for your foot while it's still clipped in. In general, this is a good thing for injury reduction; however, many elite riders prefer less float so that all of their energy goes directly to the pedal.

When setting your seat height, get into a stand and have someone watch you. With your feet clipped into the pedals and your foot at the bottom of the stroke (closest to the ground) and parallel to the ground (don't point your toes), your knee should be nearly fully extended, with just a slight bend. When you turn the pedals as if you are riding, imagine a metal rod through your hips. That rod should stay parallel to the ground all the way through your pedal stroke.

When you are out riding in a group, look for that person whose hips are rocking back and forth as they ride along. This is how you know their seat is too high (and why they'll have a terrible rash at the end of the ride).

Bike Tip #3

Fixed (non-rotating) weight reduction is overrated. Most riders carry more excess weight in fat than they can shave off their bikes; save your money.

For all but the very best riders, shaving a few grams of weight (particularly on parts that don't spin) is a waste of money. You will often feel pressure to spend money on titanium and carbon-fiber parts (or whole new bikes) to reduce your bike weight in tiny increments. At shops, fellow riders will say, "Dude, my bike only weighs thirteen and a half pounds. What is yours, like eighteen, man?" But run this test before you do anything else: reach down towards your belly button and grab a hunk of flesh. If that weighs more than the part you are going to replace, work on that weight instead, and save the money to buy good quality food.

If you *want* to spend money on your bike to reduce weight, start with things that spin. Weight reduction in wheels, pedals, gears, and cranks will have the most impact on your performance.

Bike Tip #4

The quality of your bike shorts makes a huge difference. Don't scrimp on them, or you will suffer. There are tons of choices when it comes to shorts, and this is *not* the item to bargain-hunt for. Lousy stitching will chafe you and poor-quality material won't last more than a few washes. Consider the shape of the pad; pay attention to what it's made of and its thickness. These elements have a big impact on comfort. The number of panels refers to the number of shaped fabric pieces that make up the short; more is typically better. Money-conscious me wore a low-end bicycle short one year on the Melon Patch Tour, and after seventy miles, I was reformed. I won't ride with anything but Sugoi now.

Bike Tip #5

The 169-gram torture saddle makes your bike cool, but doesn't make it faster; pain reduces focus and effort in most humans.

I have seen and sold bike seats that look like medieval torture devices. When your bike is in the rack at the transition area it will look really intimidating with that sleek carbon plate and no padding, but when your ass hurts so bad that you hobble like a bull rider during the run, I will come trotting by with a smile on my face.

A seat is fixed weight. It means almost nothing in terms of speed. Be comfortable.

Bike Tip #6

Tire pressure is huge for minimizing flats and reducing effort. Buy a good floor pump and use it before you ride, every time. Many flats are caused by under-inflation. If your tire doesn't have enough air and you run over a stone or a big crack in the road, the tire flattens out and the tube gets pinched against the rim, causing a puncture.

The more pressure there is in the tire, the less the tire comes in contact with the road, which decreases your rolling resistance. This means that if your tires are properly inflated, you'll go faster and work less than if they're underinflated.

Keep the tires inflated to the maximum recommended pressure for that specific tire. Some of us go a little higher than that, especially during races. It is nearly impossible to get enough pressure in your tire with a little frame-mounted hand pump; those things are just for emergencies to get you home after a flat. Buy a floor pump.

Tires lose air over time, so you'll need to re-inflate them often. Don't worry if your tire pressure drops by ten or twenty pounds when it sits in the garage for a while. This is normal, and it is not necessarily a leak. Once you become experienced, you can tell pretty well how full your tires are simply by pushing down hard on them with your thumb.

<u>Bike Tip #7</u>

Before every ride, run through this checklist: tire pressure, brake release levers closed, wheel spindles secure, helmet, sunscreen, flat kit, and emergency money. Make yourself go through a routine every time before you ride.

Most bikes (unless they belong in a museum) have a lever that opens the brake caliper up to allow you to remove or install the wheel without totally taking apart the brake. It is a really common oversight to forget to put that lever back in the closed position after repairing a flat or after taking your wheel off to fit your bike into your car. If you don't close the lever, the braking will be either really poor or not work at all. You do not want to find this out as you are heading off the road towards an embankment. Same thing goes for the wheel spindle lever, which clamps the wheel in place. Eric has nightmares that he is flying down a steep technical mountain road, and then realizes that he forgot to tighten his front wheel clamp.

You should always stick a few bucks into your saddlebag. You never know when you might need to make a call or buy a drink because your water bottle flew off when you hit a pothole.

<u>Bike Tip #8</u>

Ultra-narrow tires shave off seconds in a 40K ride, while flats add minutes. My father and Eric once lost a forty-mile bike race in Baytown, Texas, because Eric flatted out on skinny tires. Not worth the risk. I see a lot of people riding on ultrathin eighteen-millimeter tires in circumstances that don't make sense to me. Yes, these tires shave off a tiny bit of rotating weight, and arguably, they are more aerodynamic as they have a narrower profile to the wind. However, they have a higher likelihood of flatting. So over a 40K bike course, they may save the average rider ten seconds (yes, that little), but the risk is a flat.

How long does it take you to change a flat? In the best of circumstances, I can do a rear wheel in about five minutes. Eric can do it in two minutes, but then he has done it more times than I would care to count. To me, it just ain't worth it.

What really makes me chuckle, though, is when the aerodynamic argument is brought up by some huge guy with terrible body position and a too-loose jersey flapping in the breeze while he rides along on his eighteen-millimeter tires. I want to pull him aside and say, "Buddy, if you just got down in the drops once in a while and got a jersey that was the right size, it would have fifty times the positive effect that those tiny tires do."

Bike Tip #9
Riding like a fool on congested roadways hurts all of us, so if you can get to quiet roads, do it. If not, obey all traffic rules. It drives me nuts when I see a rider cranking through downtown traffic, ignoring traffic rules, sprinting like he's in the time trial of the first stage of the Tour. These people—and there are unfortunately many of them—seem to think the rules of the road don't apply to cool people like them. They act like vehicle drivers should telepathically know which road rules the cyclist is going to ignore, and be able to anticipate his reckless moves. They assume all drivers have perfect vision and don't get blinded by the sun, don't have other obstacles to avoid, and would sacrifice their vehicles to avoid hitting him.

We need drivers to like us. We need them to want to share the road when necessary. We want them to vote for legislation that helps us. We want them to agree (without protesting!) to be inconvenienced when roads are closed for our races. Some people I have talked to believe that they can ride wherever they want and as recklessly as they want to, because they think they'd only hurt themselves. *They are wrong.* They are hurting all of us by encouraging drivers to stereotype all cyclists as ignorant and selfish.

If you live in a high-traffic area, if it's at all possible, throw your bike in a car and drive somewhere where there are not as many cars, and where sharing the road is easy. At the very least, please be careful, obey the road rules, and bend over backwards to be courteous to drivers. If your normal time over your favorite route is twenty seconds slower because you braked and yielded to a turning car, it's not going to kill you. But if you don't ride that way all the time, then someday it might.

<u>Bike Tip #10</u>
Each time before you clip in, close your eyes and take a minute to thank those that make it possible for you to do what you are about to do. Most of us ride a bicycle because we want to, because we enjoy it, and because it's good for us. I have had the opportunity to travel quite a bit, and have seen conditions of hopeless abject poverty for a staggering number of people. There are people who spend their entire lives trying to scrape together enough for their families to eat that day. There are huge parts of the world with no paved roads and nowhere to ride, even if circumstances allowed it.

All of us that have the opportunity to ride are blessed and lucky. People have fought and died for the lives we live. People have worked hard, paid taxes, sacrificed and volunteered for the things we now take for granted. Service people like police officers, public works employees, fire and emergency service workers, and many others spend their days doing jobs that make our rides possible. There are people we love that are around us taking care of things in a manner that allows us the time and opportunity to do the thing we love to do. We owe a debt of gratitude. We need to always acknowledge that and keep it in our hearts. We need to stand on a soapbox and broadcast our appreciation every chance we get. We need to be grateful.

And one of the groups we should thank? The owners of your small, local bike shops. I encourage you to identify the shops in your area, visit them, talk to the staff, figure out the one where you fit in, and then support it with your business. Bike shops are not all the same, and they will not all fit your personality. Find the one that does, lock the address into your GPS, and support it with your business.

Yes, you can typically buy bikes and components for a few bucks less if you buy online, but every time you click "add to cart," you are pounding a nail in the coffin of your local shop. There will be times when you'll need to run out and get a tube for that ride in the morning, and if we do not make good choices, that shop will not be there. The margins on bikes are very, very small, and with the increasing business going to the internet "stores," margins and volumes have also shrunk dramatically on the accessories that used to keep the shops alive.

You can still contribute to the Eric Hutchins Bicycle Shop Ownership Recovery Fund. Make the check payable to Pamela Fagan Hutchins, please.

THIS SHOULD LEAD TO A
SPIKE IN ICY HOT SALES.

It's amazing the stupid things a smart woman sometimes does. Like me, for example. I took a two-month exercise hiatus in the midst of what was supposed to be the initial stage of training for the MS 150 bicycle race. Instead, I pounded out rewrites on two books and wrote the first draft of a third.

My main source of exercise that year had been bicycling because of the plantar fasciitis I had in my foot. I had found that my (excuse me for bluntness here, but it's about to get much worse anyway) crotch is my bicycling Achilles heel. About the only time it doesn't hurt to ride a bike is when I've put enough miles on it to achieve the consistency of old shoe leather. Any break in the training routine, and rawhide turns to flannel. Not good. Two months off is definitely a significant break.

So Eric and I hopped on the bikes the week after I completed my writing sprint. The ride went fine for a while, but, as expected, my nether region failed first. The next day I had abraded areas—not scabs, per se, and certainly not open wounds, but *scabbish* and *openish*. Technically, the areas of interest were east and west of the crotch. Underneath, I was bruised. So, I thought a little topical relief was in order. I recalled the awesome soothing capabilities of Aspercreme.

"Eric, do we have Aspercreme for my hoochie coochie?" I asked.

"You're not supposed to use it anywhere near your hoochie coochie." His tone of voice implied I was a lovable yet simple creature with an IQ of thirty-seven. I assumed, by force of will, that he wasn't patronizing me, and I responded rationally.

"Well, I'm not putting it *on* my hoochie, more like an inch or two away."

"Pamela, this is a bad idea." He flipped the channels, looking for the Arizona Cardinals. Obviously, it was not *his* crotch in extreme distress.

I went in search of Aspercreme. I couldn't find any. But I did find Icy Hot, which I was pretty sure was the same thing, although I'll admit I didn't read the directions all that well, because it was dark. We ride the bikes on our indoor training stands with the lights off in the living room while we watch football or old TV series, and Eric was already riding. So, ever so carefully, I applied the Icy Hot only in the exact non-hoochie areas that hurt.

"Eric, it feels fine." I hopped on the bike and started pedaling. My little bruisey areas began to feel hot. The warming sensation was quite pleasant and the pain eased.

"I'm rockin', honey, but actually this Icy Hot is slightly more hot than icy," I said. The warming sensation spread. It grew hotter. Suddenly, the careful, limited topical application migrated. Once it started, it went viral.

"OH MY GOD!" I hollered.

"What now?" Eric ~~sighed~~ asked lovingly.

"It's like somebody stuck a hot poker up my vajayjay!!"

"There are so many things I could say right now, but I'll restrain myself."

"The Icy Hot is crawling up my personal parts, and you're making a joke."

"What did the directions say?"

"'Not near mucous membranes.' But it's not like I stuck it up my nose."

"Maybe it ought to say, 'Hey Pamela, that means not within two inches of any orifice, including but not limited to your hoochie.'"

"Exactly. But it didn't. Shame on them."

We rode in semi-silence, the only sound my occasional moans. But you know what? That damn stuff worked. My you-know-what hurt so bad that I didn't notice my bruisey spots at all anymore.

Kids, don't try this at home. Oh, and before anyone panics on my behalf, I did not sustain any permanent injuries in this incident.

IT'S NOT (JUST) ABOUT THE BIKE.

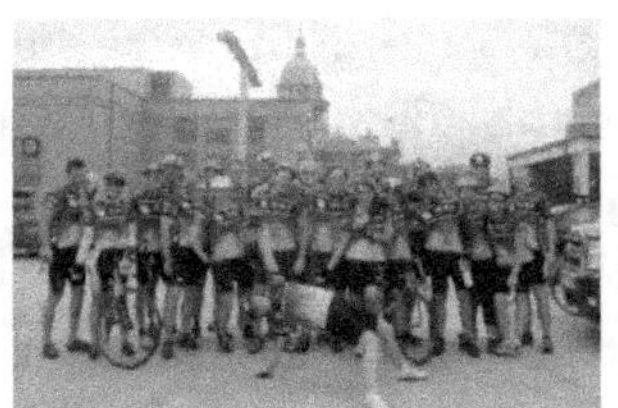

Hey, y'all, we rode with Team MRE in the BP MS 150—which, that year, was the MS 175 for us—and it rocked!!!! Day one from Houston to LaGrange we rode one hundred miles, and day two we did the La Grange to Austin leg of seventy-five miles. My butt took on a semi-permanent bicycle-seat shape. Ouch.

Funniest memories of the weekend? My husband coming out of the first rest stop porta-john bemoaning his Oakley sunglasses in the poo, followed by my husband coming out of the second rest stop porta-john bemoaning his water bottle in the poo. Oops.

His favorite memory, though, is probably moi exiting a porta-john with my stretchy thong underwear (no seams = no painful chafing) pulled up and over the back of my shirt, where they had hooked on my iPhone in my back shirt pocket. I did not realize that I had hooked said undies in this delightful T-fashion a whole six inches up my back until I tried to access the iPhone. Bicyclists will understand that the affected parts are in so much pain from the bike seat by this point that a little wedgie is nothing you'd notice. My oops.

Favorite cycling wear? Bicycle pants with the words "Mighty Fine" printed right above the butt region. Bicycling sleeves in flesh-colored fabric with tattoos. And cheetah pants. My least favorite? My own bubble-baboon-butt bike shorts covered by bubble-baboon-butt bicycle leggings on Sunday. Someone took a picture of my double ass. Hideosity.

Best part of the ride? The trip through Bastrop State Park on the challenge course. So gorgeous, and so much harder than anyone had told me. Hello, can you say, "I didn't walk my bicycle up a single one of those bitchin' hills like so many of the men I saw and passed"? Pink bikes rock! First runner-up for fave part was the area around Fayetteville, for the terrain and off-the-hook wildflowers. Wow.

Drunkest team finish? MRE! We met at Mi Madre's Restaurant in Austin Sunday afternoon—with a margarita machine—until all our team members had assembled, then rode one more mile to the finish as a team. Some people had been at Mi Madre's since 11:43 in the morning . . . we rode the finish at 3:00. Uh oh. Eric and I don't drink, so it was even funnier to us. And we finished at 12:30, so we got to watch a lot of funny. At one point, I heard a teammate asking, "Has anybody seen my beaver?" OK, I am exaggerating the drunkenness just a little. That woman was riding with a stuffed beaver on her handlebars.

Things I never want to hear again? Guys with too much testosterone bellowing "on your left!" as they pass by ten feet away. Yes, dude, I know you're passing me. I'm still gonna kick your ass on my pink bike by the time the day is through, when you're lounging around on break and I'm powering through. What-evuh.

Our sponsor, MRE Consulting, put their top fundraisers (yes, that included us) up in a hotel in Brenham, fed us all weekend, and matched our pledges dollar for dollar. Übercaptain Matt Welch made Everything More Fun.

Not only did my husband and I ride together on our pink and blue bikes the whole way without me indulging in a single ugly mood swing, even on the last hill in the park, but four of our five children met us at the finish on day two, and our Longhorn daughter brought homemade cookies. And three of the four wanted to ride with us next year. Well, that's the second best thing.

The very best thing, hands down, was that we raised $5,200 for multiple sclerosis and got to see some of the inspiring and wonderful people who work harder battling that disease every day than we ever do out enjoying ourselves on bicycles.

Yep, tears at the finish, both days. This was way more than a training ride.

THE HOMING PIGEON

When we first got together, my husband made some brash claims:

- "I don't snore"—the man revs up like a weed eater every night;

- "I'll be finished in fifteen minutes"—always means an hour;

- "I'm absolutely positive this is going to work"—translates roughly to "I'm pretty sure if I work on this for six more years I'll find a partial solution";

- "Pigs are my favorite animals"—substitute whatever animal he is currently looking at or dreaming of installing in our backyard; and my personal favorite . . .

- "I'm a frickin' homing pigeon."

Let me tell you, the one thing he most decidedly is *not* is a homing pigeon. Usually, for the sake of his tender feelings, we pretend to (sort of) believe him. But recently Eric may have convinced even himself of the fallacy of his claim. Or maybe not.

Eric and I had gone on a bicycle ride in central Houston on the concrete path along Brays Bayou on a gorgeous spring Sunday. However, Eric wanted to go further and faster than me, so we parted after ninety minutes. As he pedaled off, he assured me he'd be home in another hour and a half, in time to go to the Houston Livestock Show and Rodeo on a "double date," at the request of his seventeen-year-old daughter Liz and her boyfriend. (Ah, weren't they sweet to ask us to go with them? Don't you dare ask who paid!)

Eric did not make it home in an hour and a half. Two hours rolled by and Liz and I were nervous—she, about getting to the rodeo; me, about my husband who had a history of wicked bicycle wrecks. No word from Eric, despite our repeated texts.

Just as I was about to go out looking for him in the car, the door burst open.

"Sorry sorry sorry sorry, I know I'm late, but I got just a little tiny bit lost." In galloped Eric on his smurf-blue ~~figure skates~~ bicycle shoes that matched his bobble-head blue helmet. (He picked out the shoes, but the helmet was my bad matchy-match choice. Sorry, love!)

Liz and I looked at each other. At least one of us rolled her eyes.

He went on, breathless, fast-talking. "I ended up south of 610, somehow."

"What?!?" I spit the word out so hard that I think I splattered him with saliva. Woops. Luckily, he didn't notice; his face was already beaded with sweat.

But his locational announcement was huge. Folks, Eric was riding on a bike path alongside a bayou. In Houston, our bayous are concrete aqueducts fifty feet deep and one hundred and fifty feet across. Kinda hard to stray *five miles through city traffic* south of a bike path alongside a bayou, and not even notice. Plus, the path is on the north side of the bayou. How in the hell did he get *across* the water? Did he sprout wings from his bum and fly?

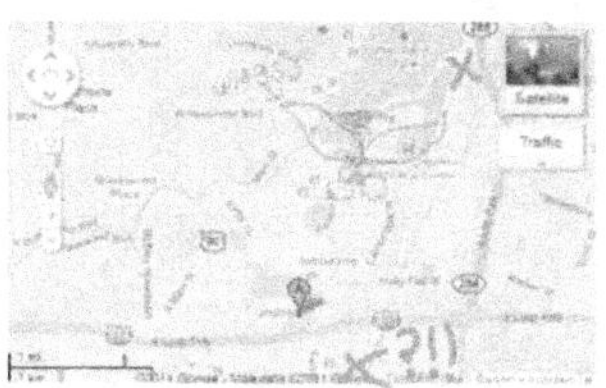

See map, above: Eric was supposed to be at the north X, but crossed water and an interstate to end up at the south X. Note smurf cyclist with butt wings hovering over map—could that be him?

He tried to explain. "There was construction around the medical center. I got confused. I guess I crossed the bayou somehow. The first time I knew I was off the path was when I turned my head at a red light and saw the medical center in the distance. So I looked around and saw I was southwest of Reliant Stadium [home of the Houston Texans football team, in case you're wondering]."

Normally, this would be funny but not a big deal. But during Rodeo at Reliant Center, traffic is insane and the drivers are frustrated, which makes it very dangerous for a bicyclist.

"It's a miracle you're alive," I said.

"I was pretty nervous about the traffic a few times." This was a big admission from Eric. He'd nearly died five years before in a head-on collision with a car, which wasn't even the first time that had happened to him.

"How'd you find your way home? Did you cut across on Bellfort?" I asked.

"Nah, I didn't want to get any further lost. I retraced my path to the bayou."

I just shook my head back and forth in a "no, I didn't marry a man who is such a danger to himself" motion. Thank God, they marked the route on the Hotter'N Hell Hundred each year, or he'd end up in Canada instead of Wichita Falls.

"Um, Dad, can you, like, hurry so we can go to the rodeo?" Liz asked. Our kids tend to hide their concern for us well.

Eric nodded as he took off his cycling shoes and headed to the shower. He couldn't help one last salvo, however. "Think how lost I would have been if I didn't have my homing pigeon instincts."

Homing pigeon, my ass. At least I know he'll always need me, if for nothing other than directions.

LOVE ME, LOVE MY FEET.

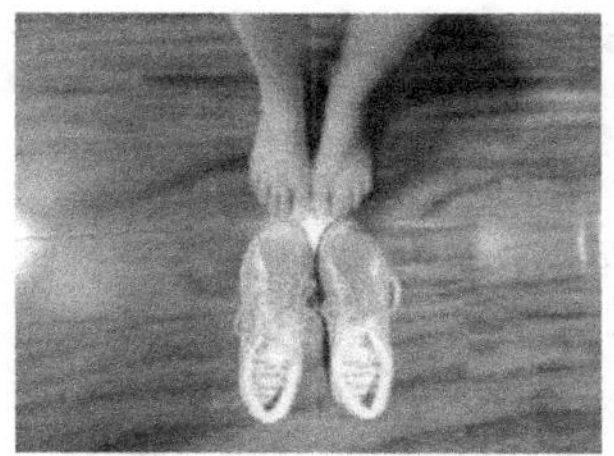

Eric loves me. He really, really loves me. I know this because at least once a week, he massages my feet for an hour and a half. Not fifteen minutes. Not an hour. A full one and a half hours.

My feet aren't hideous, but they aren't the prettiest part of me, either. I have at least two black toenails in a state of perpetual death from running. All my toes shed layers from their tips each week due to their captivity in running shoes in humid Houston. The cracks in my heels are as deep as the cracks in the dirt around our drought-ravaged and water-rationed yard. I walk around barefoot more than I should on floors swept and mopped less than is ideal, leaving a dark stain on the bottom of my feet with little fuzzies and pebbles clinging to my skin. Unless I've just showered, I've probably either recently been immersed in chlorine or had on a pair of running or (worse) biking shoes, so my dogs always have a distinctive aroma.

Eric doesn't mind. He rubs them anyway. He buys special creams and lotions to try on them. He endures sitting positions that are hell on his contorted vertebra, the one that he refuses to have fusion on, because he can take the pain.

I love Eric. I really, really love Eric. So I *let* him massage my feet. I suffer through one and a half hours of excruciating pain as he digs his thumbs deep into my tight arches that are crunchy with scar tissue. I bite my lip to keep from begging him to stop when he trenches up the sides of my aching Achilles tendons. I manage to hold still even if he works the knots, the knots he finds where none should be, leaving angry blue-green-black bruises behind, because I can take the pain.

He loves me. He wants me to triathlon with him. And I love him. I love bicycling and running and to be with my husband. We both hate the plantar fasciitis that kept me runless for eighteen months. So, I stretch and stretch and stretch and stretch and stretch. I've tried a million expensive therapies that didn't work, and twice that many wraps and shoe inserts. I wear Strassberg socks on both feet some nights. I roll my arches on oh-so-hard golf balls. I don über-goofy compression socks for my runs. I rock VFFs and Newtons instead of traditional running shoes.

And Eric massages my feet. Because he loves me. And because without those massages, he'd be short one Half Ironman training partner. But mostly because he loves me.

ICE CREAM CAUSES MURDER, AND OTHER MYTHS

I love statistics. For instance, did you know that the more ice cream that's sold in a city, the higher the murder rate there is? Does this mean murderers like ice cream? That ice cream causes murders? Or just that both occur more in warm-weather months? Hmmmmm. Be careful how you link your stats.

Consider the article linking up stats here: *The Barefoot Running Injury Epidemic {http://running.competitor.com/2010/05/features/the-bare foot-running-injury-epidemic_10118}*. The author posits that people who switch to "barefoot" or Vibram FiveFingers running sustain more injuries than people who run in traditional running shoes. Read the whole article and you'll see that it's hard to draw this conclusion in the first place. But also consider all the information not included in the article:

- Successful transition from non-barefoot to barefoot running is dependent on completely changing *form*.

- Running barefoot with the same form used with high wedge/high structure running shoes is a recipe for disaster.

- Runners are advised to switch over to barefoot running gradually, to build the underdeveloped support muscles in the feet, ankles and calves that will be called to action by the new running form.

I developed plantar fasciitis while running in highly-structured Adidas adiStar running shoes that forced my foot into a heel-strike position, and then I didn't run for more than a year while I let myself heal. I have tried numerous therapies and exercises, and I will tell you what has worked for me. I rested my foot for months. I stretched. I stretch and stretch and stretch and stretch and stretch my plantar and my Achilles. For a few months, I taped my foot for walking. I wore the Strassberg sock at night, although I know some people swear by the plantar fasciitis boot instead. I changed my running form and took up minimalist running wearing VFFs and Newtons. I switched to shifting my weight forward onto my toes and NEVER NEVER NEVER letting my heels touch the ground.

The two orthopedists I visited were almost completely worthless, except for making the diagnosis. "Do nothing," they said. Wrong answer. "Do something," my heart cried, so I did. I healed, and then I changed my game so that I wouldn't reinjure myself. No more highly-structured, heel-striking shoes for me.

I love statistics; I find them entertaining. But I love using my own brain even more.

PEACE OUT

Peace doesn't always flow like a river at our house. Between kid drama, puppy drama, work, finances, and health issues, peacelessness sometimes dams up the waterway and creates a dark lake of ugh.

Eric and I were tri-training. My foot had healed, and we were ramping back up. Then Eric learned he had an infected, abscessed tooth that would need another root canal when the antibiotics had done their work. My friends warned me that infections of the teeth are potentially quite serious, and can impact the heart, the brain, and other organs. My friends turned out to be right.

After the first round of antibiotics, Eric's fever and health were worse, not better. His endodontist started him on a stronger antibiotic and punted Eric to an oral surgeon, who couldn't get him in for two weeks. In the meantime, the endodontist didn't tell Eric not to run—possibly because he didn't know that running had been elevating Eric's pulse recently. (I suspect there was also some *crafting* of the report Eric gave me about his restrictions.)

We went for a training run together a few nights after he started the new meds, and from the get-go, my super-fit husband had tremendous difficulty. After two miles, he was drunkenish, weaving, staggering a bit, glazy-eyed. Our pace was middlin'-turtle already, and

I knew I had to make him walk. But only a fool would tell Eric to stop mid-effort.

I did that once, during the Hotter'N Hell Hundred bicycle race in Wichita Falls a few years ago, when Eric succumbed to dehydration caused by a stomach constriction that he later had corrected. He lurched around at a rest stop, catching the eye of an on-site physician, who managed with my assistance to wrangle Eric under the tent for an examination. Fifteen minutes later, he released Eric and I helped him finish the race—a first in our athletic partnership, believe me. Normally I'm the parasite and Eric is the strong, healthy carrier.

I had not used my powers since. I know well that Eric hates to stop. He feels exercise is critical to his physical and mental health, and his stress had mounted to peak levels in the past two months. His youngest daughter had left for college, his stomach procedure and then this mystery illness had made it difficult to work out, and he was still undergoing pain treatments and epidurals for his back, which was broken in a bike wreck in 2006. He was never able to fit every-thing he wanted to do into a day, and frankly, he felt like crap and hadn't dared to admit it. The weight of it all was crushing his usually ebullient spirit.

So, how could I get him to stop running without making a bad situation explosive? I slowed to a walk and made a dramatic show of scratching mosquito bites. Eric slowed with me.

"Are you ready to restart?" he asked, in a spot-on imitation of Johnny Depp à la *Pirates of the Caribbean*.

"Welllllllll . . . my feet really hurt. I've been slacking off for five weeks, and this distance is too much for them. Gotta be smart, build them back up. I'll have to walk." When in doubt, blame it on the plantar fasciitis. Hopefully the darkness between the widely-spaced streetlights on the bayou path was heavy enough to hide the lie on my face.

Without a word he fell in beside me, holding my hand and unable to talk further. He stumbled along. We took a shortcut home. Fifteen minutes later he was no better, so he took his blood pressure: fifty percent higher than usual, and it's borderline high on a good day. That night, it was scary high.

I put him in bed with a cold cloth on his forehead and snuggled in beside him, stroking his face and considering forcing him to go to the emergency room. Eric admitted that his jaw hurt, and his sinuses now hurt, too. (The x-rays of his abscessed tooth had shown that the infection had eaten a hole in his jaw and was marching on to his sinus cavities.) We compromised: if his blood pressure came down significantly in half an hour, he'd contact his endodontist, let him know of the worsening situation, ask for a different antibiotic, and enlist his help in moving the oral surgery sooner. His pressure came down just enough that he made it through the night.

The next morning Eric said he felt passable, and promised to call the endodontist first thing, but I knew he wouldn't. I contacted his primary care physician, none other than my father. Dr. Dad suggested in strong terms that I make it clear to the oral surgeon the time had come to do something.

I pinged Eric.

"Too busy," he said, snappish.

"Give me the number."

"Don't have it."

"Give me the name."

He complied, and gave me a list of days he couldn't go. Then he caved. "I'll go today if they can get me in."

I love him. I understood. I was scared, too.

The endodontist's office responded beautifully, despite my fear that they would dismiss a hysterical wife. Maybe the tremor in my voice as I explained my fears about my husband's general health and heart condition helped. They paged the oral surgeon to let her know that it was an emergency, and the surgeon's assistant moved the procedure up to four days later. Progress.

The assistant interrupted my gushing thank yous to say, "Hold please, it's the surgeon again."

I held for mere seconds.

"Can he go right now? They looked at his films, and the surgeon is clearing her schedule for him. But he has to go now."

"I'll get him there." I left out the "if I have to drag his bloody carcass behind me on a travois" part, but it was implied.

And that is how it came to pass that my husband—who finally accepted that he should worry and obey—ended up with a swollen face and a jaw packed with bovine bone three hours later. Thank God for that hyper-responsive surgeon. The culprit for months of undisclosed pain and illness? A hairline crack in his tooth that was too tight to appear on x-rays, but formed a perfect superhighway for bacteria into his jaw tissue.

"Well?" I asked as I bustled him back out to the car.

Through a mouthful of gauze, Eric conveyed in the strongest possible terms that he never wanted to hear his jawbone scraped again. (Why he chose to remain awake is a mystery to me.) The doctor told him she was optimistic that she had removed all the infected tissue, and that her topical antibiotic was strong enough to deal with what was left behind, but she also kept Eric on oral antibiotics. He was by turns jubilant and chastened, relieved and grateful.

"I ahmrave ahrmto ahrmgo ahrmback," he said. Or tried to.

Translation: besides a normal follow-up about the infection and wound site, he'd been ordered to get another round of bone grafts in January, a metal plate in April, and a new tooth installed the next summer. Plus the follow-up with his cardiologist ASAP. Worse things have happened to nice people, I know, but he was bummed.

Yet in the midst of all this noise was love. Me. The kids. His parents. *Me.*

When we married, Eric had said his greatest goal for our new life was peace. Mind you, he had an overflowing extra-large Samsonite rolling case full of goals that weighed against the possibility of him ever finding it, but what he longed for, now that he had love, was a strife-free zone. A center. A stillness. A safe place to curl up by the fire, legs stretched out, head back, hot chocolate with homemade whipped cream on top in hand. I had promised to give him that. Yeah, me. The one who is a bit, well, mercurial.

But life doesn't allow for perfect peace. You have to find your peace amidst the unceasing chaos of bills, illnesses, injuries, work, heartbreaks, and crises. Eric had lost his peace. He had just flat-out lost it. I had failed to give it to him, too. From where he stood, that day was yet another in the latest long list of examples of peace escaping him.

And I empathized. I'd had my own run of less-than-peaceful, with the hormones, the ITBS, the plantar fasciitis, and life in general. I didn't know how to fix it for either of us, just like I didn't know for sure how to fix his tooth, or even how to make him stop running, but I was trying. I wanted to figure it out, and I wanted to help him find that chimera, that life without turmoil. Or at least find peace within it. So I ran out while he was in surgery and gathered up a few gifts, hoping they would be the electric paddles that would shock his heart into accepting peace in the here and now.

We got into our crusty old Suburban and Eric opened the gifts. And maybe it was the drugs, maybe it was his jacked-up emotions, but his tears rolled. I helped him put the very manly leather necklace on, to nestle the tiny *E*, *Peace*, and *P* in his thirteen chest hairs against his gigantic heart. It hung out of sight under his shirt, warmed by his skin. I'd waited six years to do this—to replace the gold chain he'd worn since childhood, but that I hated because it was a reminder of the pasts without each other that we had agreed to leave behind.

He held the heavy distressed wooden block with the word "Peace" on it that I hoped he would put in his office, and he read aloud the card that anchored the two gifts:

Peace. It does not mean to be in a place where there is no noise, trouble, or hard work. It means to be in the midst of those things and still be calm in your heart.

I love this card more than I can express. Eric seemed to, too. And that moment felt like the safest time to confess my subterfuge on the previous night, when I had stopped his run. He groaned.

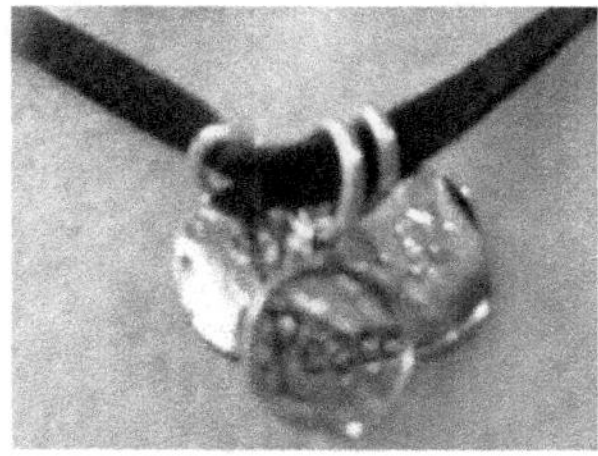

Above: E-Peace-P

"I promise to use my powers only for good, never for evil," I said. "But I love you, and hear me loud and clear on this: I won't let you harm yourself."

His nod was barely perceptible, but he did nod.

TAN LINES

I have been threatening a scandalous exposé about my husband, and the time has come. The following is an actual conversation between us.

"Honey, you look like one of those double-stuffed Oreos from the back, except you're milk chocolate instead of dark chocolate," I said.

Eric shot me a look over his shoulder. Not an appreciative-of-his-wife's-sense-of-humor kind of look.

"Whaaatttt?" he asked.

"You know, baby, your tan lines. From swimming."

In the summer, Eric swims at noon two to three days a week, outside. He wears knee-length jammers, and the good Lord blessed him with fast-tanning olive skin. I love holding hands with him when his fingers are like the latte and mine are the steamed-milk topping.

"Very funny. Don't write about that." He hopped into the shower.

"Oh, I wouldn't write about that. If I did, people would be thinking about your naked hiney."

"Exactly."

"Yep."

"So, to be clear, you are promising me you won't write about my tan lines?"

"That's what I'm saying. I think people would be *offended* if I wrote about it. Children might see it."

"OK. Good. Thanks."

"Yup. You're welcome. But I'm not doing it for you. I'm doing it for my readership."

"Whatever, just as long as I don't see some picture of my naked ass that you took as I ran from the shower some day."

"As if. I have scruples, you know."

My appreciation for said unclothed posterior is well known in our family. One day I accidentally texted about my appreciation to his then-twenty-one-year-old daughter, who forever more has called him Sweet Cheeks and Honey Buns. She gets a kick out of it. Him, not so much.

I keep telling him it could be much worse. At least I really, really like him.

"What if I didn't like you, and I wrote about *that*?" I asked him once.

"What if you didn't write about me at all?"

"Then you wouldn't know whether I liked you or not!"

"It's a risk I would be willing to take."

I don't think he really means it. So, anyway, I just thought y'all would enjoy the photo below.

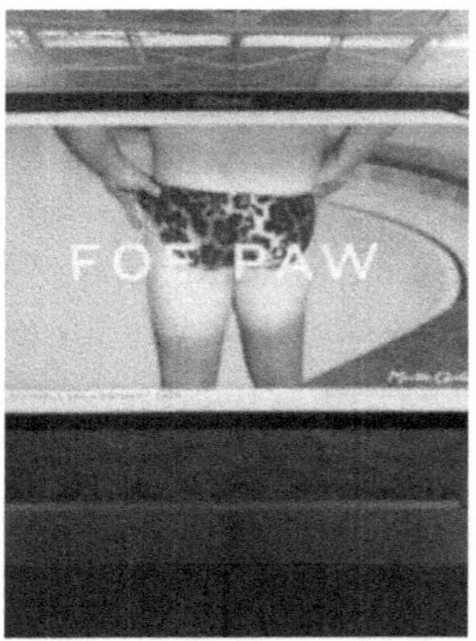

Above: Photo taken of LCD advertisement at Hobby Airport in Houston

No, this is not actually Eric's butt. His is *at least* ten times better;

he may be a year or two past twenty-seven, but he is a workout fiend, which is not without its benefits. This is exactly what his tan lines look like, though. And he does have this bathing suit.

Meow.

Kidding. Of course he does not have *this* bathing suit . . . but pictures do exist of him in a Speedo, and the ever-present threat of me publishing them through the interwebs hangs like a guillotine over him. There's a reason he's so nice to me: fear.

BOOGIE SHOES

I am blessed with the love of good friends. Some of them I've never even met, but thanks to the power of the internet and the bond of writers, we hang out virtually. We chill. We share. We bond. We give presents.

My writer friend Heidi upped the ante one year with a present she knew would rock my world: a ballroom dance lesson for Eric and me. We went, we sucked, and we loved it so much we bought more. Or, rather, we pooled my gift bounty and a bunch of nice people made it possible for us to buy more with their generous checks and such.

You would think two Half-Ironman triathletes would find dancing a breeze, but we learned on day one that this dancing shit will wear you O-U-T. I glowed, and Eric sweated like a pig. His face was as red as when I write about his Speedo, seriously. An hour of rumba transformed me from Pamelot to Puffalot.

And our instructors are like freakin' drill sergeants (which I can appreciate, as the family disciplinarian). They won't even let us *talk* to each other. Or drop our arms—excuse me, our *frame*. Or look at our feet. Or stop if we mess up. Or wear street shoes. It's like we're training for the dorky-white-couple dance-Olympics or something.

. . .

ABOVE: Our suede-bottomed fairy shoes.

So, as you can tell—extreme physical exercise + rigid discipline—it's totally our type of thing! We had five lessons left, and after that they wanted us to pay like, oh, a mere trifle for fifteen more lessons. A mere trifle as in fifteen hundred **smackers**. Yes, you read that right. And with me fresh out of gift money, too.

Five to go . . . could we become proficient in that amount of time? And by that, I don't mean ready for *Dancing with the Stars*, but just good enough that Eric doesn't yell the F word on the dance floor (which we learned is perfectly all right with our instructors, as long as we are safely practicing in their studio) more than once every ten minutes.

So we asked.

OH NO, the studio manager said. No, we could not make you social dancers in such a short time.

We gritted our teeth. Oh yeah, buddy? Just watch us.

So we hatched a plan. Instead of just squeezing in a lesson, we would only go to a lesson if it was adjacent to a free (as in totally without monetary cost) group lesson, and we would attend henceforth all the free parties the studio threw to addictify its unsuspecting clientele, until we ran out of lessons.

Last Friday we took Liz, her boyfriend, Susanne, and her friend Annie to a free sock hop. {And I wore Liz's poodle skirt, y'all!} Only no one else was there when we got there! So they gave us a free group lesson. And then other people showed up, so we had the party after all. We'd been stuck on waltz, rumba, tango, and swing up until then, but that night we burst out after our free salsa lesson into the merengue and cha-cha, too. Hear us roar! We took turns dancing with the kids. Everyone had a grand time. And guess what? Eric didn't say the F word a single time.

Armed with our newfound confidence, I jumped onto iTunes and for only $45, I bought whole albums of ballroom dancing music. We put on our little fairy shoes. We folded our ping-pong table and pushed the weight bench and treadmill back against the wall in our game room. We turned on our music and we DANCED.

So. We're leaving now for our free group lesson and our expensive private lesson. Ready to milk every drop of knowledge out of these high-priced instructors {If you actually met our dance instructor, you would think I was on crack. He is probably the nicest, funniest guy in the world. He can't help it that his boss is the aforementioned drill sergeant (with too much hair gel) and the cost of their program requires a second mortgage. We love you, Alex.}. Because come hell or high water, we are going to be socially acceptable dancers when we finish this program. So there.

A FULL MOON

I spoke too soon on the triathlon training schedule, began to hope too soon about our long-awaited next Half Ironman. Because my hormones came back. Well, actually they flared up periodically. So, a few times a year, the staff at Hotze increased my progesterone, and I stayed one step ahead of the werewolf.

But in the last few months, the process had sped up. (I promise, I'm getting to a point sometime soon—Half Ironman, Pamela, you were talking about training for a Half Ironman.) It started with sleeping problems—exhaustion/insomnia/exhaustion/insomnia and so on. Then, more three a.m. night sweats. Next, the migraines and carb cravings shot up—my kingdom for an apple fritter!—and so did my weight.

One day I woke up and realized I felt sad; melt into the Earth sad. My hormones are raging beasts, not depressed ones, so WTH? My cycle shortened from twenty-eight days to seventeen. My breasts swelled up like angry cantaloupes. (And angry cantaloupes are really really . . . hell, I don't know, I couldn't think of anything but cantaloupes, so maybe I have the first angry cantaloupe breasts in the history of the world, but run with it—the big fat suckers are pissed off, OK?)

Other body parts wanted in on the "beat the crap out of Pamela" game. So my urethra contributed recurrent UTIs. And every injury

I'd had in the last ten years—all the old healed-up ones—rose from the dead and zombie-marched through my body. Old hamstring pull on right thigh? Torturous. A right groin strain from a few years ago? It was like I'd stabbed myself with a butter knife that lodged and slowly rotated on its own. My left shoulder, the proud bearer of a "snuggling" injury from 2007 (ye-es, a snuggling injury—we had to change sleeping positions, and it took months to heal)? So painful I cannot do any of my normally easy arm and shoulder stretches. This wacked-out muscle memory, this macabre parade of old wrongs against my body, made no sense and was crazy as hell, but it was real.

The unimpacted parts of me? My heart and lungs. If I could somehow make it, stiff-legged, through the burning tree trunks portion of my run (two or more miles), then I would burst out of my stumbling body like a butterfly from its chrysalis and I soar.

Sometimes I didn't make it past the first half mile.

The constant of my period with cramps and an accompanying UTI decreased my bicycling enthusiasm. During one ride, the pain was so intense that I did something I'd never done before: I pulled over to the side of the road and stood with my bicycle for forty-five minutes while Eric went and got the car.

And swimming? Between the migraines (which come with nausea) and the immobile shoulder, no way.

Did any of this mean I *couldn't* train? Of course not. But when you added these things to my bone-melting sadness and exhaustion, training was not appealing. Training was thus not happening very frequently. I was weak. I was ashamed.

"Sounds like menopause," a friend said.

From her mouth to my doctor's ear. The doctor I wanted to string up by her ankles. While that sounds a little extreme, I was FEELING a *lot* extreme.

I didn't want to get my hopes up too far that the end was near. And yet I needed some hope. I hoped against hope that my hope would be rewarded. I hoped that all of this *stopped*. Either by nature or knife—I wasn't and am not above begging for a hysterectomy, y'all.

In the meantime, I had to get a grip on this. I couldn't float and fail. I had to go forth with purpose and a *plan*, a wonderful beautiful marvelous plan, even if I ended up in the same place. Here is what I came up with:

I made sure to eat more menopause-friendly foods: soy milk, blueberries, bananas, multi-grains, turkey, fish, yogurt, and cranberry juice IN; sugar, fats, and simple carbs OUT. I think I was also supposed to lay off the coffee, but hell-to-the-no. I don't drink alcohol, so nothing to give up there.

I scaled back on the intense exercise and did more walking, hiking, stretching, and weightlifting. I thought that if I took the pressure off that every workout had to live up to a "personal best" on the long march to Ironman, I would do something instead of nothing.

I started the year with doctor's appointments to rule out any other (unlikely) issues, followed by a check-in with the Hotze center. Hotze to the rescue, yay! They definitely helped, even if it didn't eliminate the problem completely.

I searched for the world's best natural sleep aid. I settled on Somnapure.

I deliberately reduced my schedule. I couldn't do it all. I had to tell myself no. Or at least maybe.

Yeah, I spent some days crying in the corner. I wanted to be Pamela again. I wanted to be an Ironwoman.

FOURTEEN GOING ON FORTY-FOUR

I love those experiences that take me back to an old moment in a heartbeat, erasing decades and all that came with them—bills, perimenopause, kids, injuries, jobs, exes, cellulite. Songs often do that for me. Play "Urgent" by Foreigner, and I am back in Amarillo at my best friend Deborah's house, with the taste of Reese's Peanut Butter Cups lingering in my mouth. When the radio plays Three Dog Night's "Joy to the World," I hear my father sing-shout "JEREMIAH WAS A BULL FROG!" and feel the jolts bouncing the smile on my six-year-old lips as his right hand pounds the steering wheel of our brown paneled station wagon.

But visceral experiences can transport me back in time as well. A smell, a sensation, something I taste—all can open the doorway to the time machine. Like bicycling in the rain did one Friday. On Fridays, I volunteer at my kids' high school during the lunch period. My glamorous job? I sell Quiznos sandwiches as a fundraiser for the football team. Publicly, I kvetch about the impact on my schedule and writing time. Secretly, I love it.

That day, though, I had a transportation issue. Eric's Suburban was in the shop, so he had no car for a few days. I had taken a week off from work to write and needed no wheels, so he was driving my car. But I needed to get to the school to sell sandwiches.

"No problem. I'll ride my bike," I said.

"Are you sure? I could come home and get you," Eric said.

"And pick me back up an hour later? That's crazy. It's a fifteen-minute bike ride, if that long."

"It *would* really help me not to leave work twice. If you're sure."

I was sure. Mostly because my pink bicycle rocks.

On that Friday, I took extra care getting ready, so as not to embarrass the kids: I brushed my hair and changed out of my stretchy exercise clothes. I even put on a cute white sleeveless sweater and a tan-and-white seersucker skort. And I applied mascara. I almost needed a nap after all that beautification effort.

I hopped on my pink bike and rode to the school. I made it just in the nick of time, locked the bike in an illegal parking spot, and sprinted into the cafeteria, where I schlepped sub sandwiches for an hour. I enjoyed a chat with Liz, who used the occasion to ask for money. I attempted to get Clark to talk to me—or even make eye contact—to no avail. Teenagers.

Right as we finished up, a thunderstorm hit. I tried to wait it out, but the storm did not accommodate me. I mounted Ole Pink in thunder, lightning, and street-floodingly-heavy rain.

The rain claimed my hair first. *Oh well, so now it looks normal,* I thought. Next to go was my mascara. Raccoon eyes. *Not a great look, but no biggie.* The last casualty, though, was my white top, which, when paired with the hair and mascara, gave me a trailer-parky look. *Maybe no one will recognize me.*

I pedaled carefully in my sopping wet flip-flops through an inch of standing water down the edge of Rice Street. I navigated through midday motorists who could not see me, riding a full two feet into the street to avoid the deeper water in the gutters. On my right-hand side was a curb. I'll admit, I was nervous, trapped in that narrow corridor with bad traction and poor visibility. I felt like I had a red X on my back, as in, "Here I am, run me over, please—it'll give me an excuse for not finishing my rewrites!"

Riding a road bicycle in the rain is far more dangerous than riding a normal bike in the rain. My dad has rain plus road bike to thank for a broken collarbone. My bike also boasts Speedplay pedals, which made a bad situation worse that day. Imagine a lollipop stuck off the side of the pedal's crank. I normally clip my cleats into the candy part of the lollipop, but I wasn't wearing my bike shoes. I was pushing the lollipops with wet flip-flops. My feet slid off the lollipops approximately every three rotations of the pedals.

And there were other issues. (There are always *other issues* with me, according to my husband). Ole Pink's tires are slicks, the almost treadless tires preferred for speedy road bicycling. Slicks are not designed for wet roads *at all*. The brakes are caliper brakes, which are nearly worthless when they're wet. And at fifty-seven inches, my bicycle, even though it is a women-specific design with a slanted crotch post, stands on the tall side of just right. It's not easy to quickly put my feet on the ground when I have to stop.

I knew I was headed for a crash. And just as I pondered whether to indulge in a bad attitude about fate putting me on my bicycle in the rain on this road on that day, a blinding flash of memory sucked me through a vortex back to the age of fourteen, when my ten-speed Schwinn represented freedom, the freedom to fly away by myself wherever my wheels could take me.

I adored that bicycle. Suddenly I wasn't in Houston. I wasn't nearly forty-four years of age. I was almost fourteen, riding in a similar rainstorm on the way home from the Town Club swimming pool in Amarillo. The same rain landing on my face now had landed on my face thirty years before, and I had turned my face upward then to catch the big drops on my eyelashes and my tongue. I loved riding in the rain! The tires threw water up over my sandaled feet. I was soaked and delightfully cold, even though it was August. Cars had pulled over because of the storm, but not me. I was free.

And, back in the land of yesteryear, that's when it happened. The fourteen-year-old me hit a mossy spot with her front tire, the result of a constant runoff stream in the gutter from lawn-care zealots, those environmental scofflaws who water three times a day in the hottest part of the summer. The bicycle's front wheel slipped out from under me. Down I went, into the water and onto the road debris underneath.

The ground knocked the wind out of me. My right thigh and elbow took the brunt of the debris, since I had ridden on the wrong side of the road. Gravel dug tracks in my skin, leaving blood, dirt, and small rocks deeply embedded in its path. I wiped my face and the oily residue from the wet road stuck to me, stinking like a gas station. A driver honked at me and I shot her a look. *Like I fell on purpose and could move out of the way of your car if I tried, lady!* Trust me, I had serious attitude by the age of fourteen, like my own daughter does now.

I lay there for a few minutes until the pain in my elbow stinger subsided. I hoped some Good Samaritan would pick my bike and me up and give us a ride home, but no such luck. Finally, slowly, I positioned the bike and myself for a fresh start and away we pedaled, more cautiously this time.

Thirty years ago, I swore off riding in the rain. Thirty years later, here I was, riding in the rain again, in the worst of conditions and traffic.

But the memory of that fall didn't bring me fear. Instead, it brought back my love for that bicycle and the rain. It transported me to feeling young and alive, fourteen and free. I tingled all over and laughed aloud. I turned my face up to the sky and caught water in my lashes and on my tongue. I sang Eddie Rabbit's "I Love a Rainy Night" at the top of my lungs as I pedaled.

Ole Pink and I made it home upright. And I appreciated my warm shower, for sure. Even more, I appreciated my journey back in time. I smiled for the rest of the day, remembering the freedom fourteen-year-old me had to fly away on her bicycle in the rain, and the budding toughness I would nurture until it bloomed into one of my defining adult traits.

Ah, memory. In truth, I don't want to be fourteen again, although it was nice for fifteen minutes. I'd be happy to restart at thirty-four, however. I want to ride my bicycle . . . and run . . . in the rain . . .

HAPPY BIRTHDAY HALF IRONMAN

"What do you want for your birthday?" Eric asked about a week before my big double-four.

I knew exactly what I wanted. "For you to take off work and do a Half Ironman with me."

"No, seriously, what do you want?" he asked.

"Seriously, I would like you to block a day out of your midweek schedule and do a Half Ironman, just you and me. I already have it mapped out. We're in shape for it. We're feeling good. Those windows don't open for us very often. Let's jump through."

Eric requires process time. He stared at me while his brain whirled so fast I could hear the gears turning. Finally, he spoke again.

"You can't run it, Pamela. You're haven't build up enough mileage yet. You'd kill your foot."

"I don't have to run it all. I didn't last time. We can alternate walking and running, whatever feels smart once we're in the middle of it." I saw him put his hand on the open window, and I gave him a nudge. "We're both swimming and bicycling great. We'll start at the pool at 24 Hour Fitness after we drop the kids at school, then dash home to our bikes. We'll have to ride on the training stands, but our cycle computers will tell us how long to ride. Then, we'll just drive three blocks to the bayou and run 2.2-mile outs on the grass, return on the backs to the car for fuel and hydration, and repeat until we're done."

"You really are serious about this, aren't you?" He had his whole upper body through the window now, so I reached up my hand to pull him the rest of the way in.

"Real triathletes race, Eric, even if it's not on anyone else's schedule," I said, reminding him of his own words, although he certainly hadn't been talking about a home-baked non-race. "We don't know what life will dish out to us next. Let's race ourselves while we both feel good."

And so, on my forty-fourth birthday, that is exactly what we did. There were no crowds, no aid stations, and—dammit—no race t-shirts, but there were the two of us. We brought our hearts, and we brought our game. Seven hours later, we had logged roughly the same time we had three years and countless injuries ago. Yeah, I got wicked nauseous in the pool from a hormone-migraine and nearly booted, but I didn't. Yeah, we had to walk a few miles of the run to ease the impact on my foot, but so what. There were no crowds to cheer us on, but our three teenagers did manage to force out a couple of "Really? You did that today? What's wrong with you?"-type comments, which meant, "Congratulations on your excellent performance," in their own special language.

À la couples who make you want to puke, we commemorated it with a video {And, in fact, here is the video we shot in the aftermath: http://youtu.be/-RTinAArpoU.} posted to YouTube. What? You don't post your biggest life moments on YouTube? OK, maybe that's living life a little too out loud for some of you, but it fit the high of the moment.

I don't kid myself about why my husband loves me. It's because we are alike in a way that many people don't understand (or think is nuts) but that we respect. Extremes. No downtime. Pain = Awesomeness.

We celebrated—no, make that *exulted* the passage of years, the victory in the latest battle over the werewolf, the mastery of our crazy schedules and overcommitments, in our own special way. We pounded out our joy with the drumbeats of our feet. We embraced life and the living of it to the hilt. We defied aging, hormones, broken backs, farged up feet, and abscessed teeth. We found our peace, and we found our compromise between Eric's need for racing and my need for seizing the day. And we did it together. For maybe five whole minutes, we didn't talk about the next race, or when the Ironman training would start, or whether Pamela would ever get her ultra.

But you can bet we were both thinking about it. And the M-dot tattoos? 2016, baby. In the meantime, we'd just keep enjoying the craziness and pain of real life, of training and racing together.

I thought back to that long-ago family triathlon on a hot June day. I compared it to my life now and all that had transpired since. I couldn't help but smile. This. This is what I had wanted. This is what the forty-four-year-old me thought was a perfect-enough life. I didn't need youth or talent. I could live with the hormones, as long as I had this shared passion with my husband. It wasn't always easy, maybe it wasn't even normal, but to me it was perfect all the same.

EXCERPT FROM HOW TO
SCREW UP YOUR MARRIAGE

Bring me a bucket.

When people tell me and my husband that we make them want to puke, we gaze into each other's eyes and say, "Thank you!" Then we go home and make sweet, sweet love, while singing each other Marvin Gaye songs and weaving promise rings out of sea grass and clover.

It's hard work, being this nauseating. The effort involved in all this damn smiling—you wouldn't want to take it on, I promise. Totally exhausting. Add to this burden our perfect children and our perfect careers, and you've got the makings of chronic fatigue syndrome, at least.

As my youngest daughter would say, "Whatever."

The first time an acquaintance told me, "Y'all are just so cute together it makes me want to puke," I wasn't sure how to take it. It sounded like a compliment, but it felt like a barb. I thought about her sterile marriage to a nice but unaffectionate man who didn't seem to find her interesting, and about how she laughed about him behind his back. I analyzed the green look in her brown eyes; I'd seen it in other people's eyes when I was with my husband. I concluded that, given the choice, I'd like to keep my relationship over hers, thank you very much. Also, while she seemed envious in a grudgingly admiring way, I'd never seen evidence that she worked to improve her own marriage. Not once. Did she think pukeworthiness just happened by accident, by a sprinkling of pixie dust? I don't believe it does.

So, yep, I am the lucky princess with the fairytale marriage. But I'm willing to bet even Cinderella and Prince Charming had their issues. Unfortunately for my prince, I habitually and publicly confess my more interesting failings, which inevitably involve our relationship from time to time. I guess that in addition to being half of a couple who makes you want to puke, I have diarrhea of the mouth (and fingers), too. Totally irresistible, I know.

I wish I could make it sound more scintillating than it really is, maybe write about how Eric is a compulsive gambler and I am a gender-reassignment success story, and the neighbors have called the cops to break up our fights on three separate occasions. That would be exciting, but it wouldn't be true.

The truth is boring. The truth is that we are as flawed as the next couple. I adore my almost-perfect husband, who puts up with me writing about him and being a gigantic pain in the ass. I love my normal, fallible kids and stepkids {I'll refer to family members, friends, and clients from time to time. Names have been changed to protect the innocent—which Eric and I are far from.}. I love our messed-up, wacky life. But just because we adore and love each other, it doesn't mean the rest comes easily.

While I have no scandalous revelations for you, I can share the secrets of how two highly emotional, self-absorbed, over-committed Type-A losers at marriage (we are both each other's second spouse) manage our relationship into the true thing of beauty that it is.

And I do mean manage.

(Are you choking on that vomit yet? Stick around.)

If my day job counts, I am a so-called expert in human relations. As a hybrid employment attorney/human resources professional and consultant, I get paid to help grownups manage their workplace relationships. The HR principles I apply at work are, in theory, principles for humans anywhere—like humans in a marriage, even a second marriage like mine.

There's a good reason doctors don't usually treat family members:

when it comes to our loved ones, our rational selves are replaced by emotional creatures. Things get personal. Things get messy. All the psychological training in the world couldn't guarantee that someone (and by someone I mean me) will play fair.

Physician, heal thyself. HR Consultant, you too.

So it is with some embarrassment, and hopefully a bit of humility, that I will share our foibles and our feats. We understand how wrong we each got it on our first ride on the marriage-go-round, and we believe that through painful trial and error, we've finally gotten a grip on the brass ring. We know the statistics: over 40% of first marriages end in divorce and up to 67% of second do, too. The big issues—emotional intimacy, mutual support, compatibility, respect, sex, and money {And, these days, I'd have to say that technology, like social media and smartphones, makes these issues more immediate and drives up the intensity.}—get even trickier when you add stepparenting, alimony, child support, ex-spouses, and the "It's easier to say 'I quit' the second time" phenomenon. But we're beating the odds, and we want you to, as well. And so we begin. Keep your Pepto-Bismol handy.

There's nothing under the canoe, honey.

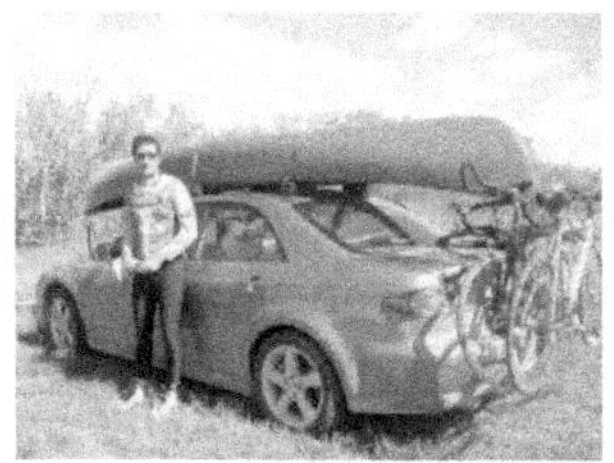

Above: This is how we roll.

My husband and I went on our honeymoon in Montana in June, which unbeknownst to us was still the dead of winter. (We hail from the Caribbean.) At the time, we were training for a Half Ironman triathlon,training for a Half Ironman triathlon, so we needed to find an upper-body strength and aerobic substitute for swimming during our two weeks of bliss. Without taking the weather into account, we'd decided that canoeing or kayaking would suffice.

So off we traipsed from Houston to Montana, where we stayed in an adorable bed-and-breakfast near Yellowstone, which we picked because the owner advertised healthy organic food. The beets, quinoa, and cauliflower kugel we were served for breakfast weren't exactly what we'd hoped for, but we felt fantastic. And hungry. Very, very hungry.

Our "Surprise! We're vegetarian!" B&B sat near a tundra lake. For those of you who have not seen a tundra lake, imagine a beautiful lake in a mountain clearing surrounded by tall evergreens. Picture deer drinking from crystalline waters, hear the ducks quacking greetings to each other as they cruise its glassy surface. Smell the pine needles in the air, fresh and earthy.

And then imagine the opposite.

A tundra lake is in the highlands, no doubt, but the similarity stops there: no trees, no windbreak, no calm surface, and no scenery. Instead, it's an ice-chunk-filled, white-capped pit of black water extending straight down to hell, stuck smack dab in the middle of a rock-strewn wasteland. Other than that, it's terrific.

Maybe it was because we were newlyweds, but somehow Eric intuited that I would love nothing more than to canoe this lake in forty-degree weather and thirty-five-mph winds, wearing sixty-seven layers of movement-restricting, water-absorbent clothing. Maybe it was because we were newlyweds, but I somehow assumed that because he knew of my dark water phobia and hatred of the cold (anything below seventy degrees), I was in good hands. My new husband assured me this lake was perfect for tandem canoeing.

So . . . we drove across the barren terrain to the lake. Eric was bouncy. I was unable to make my mouth form words other than "You expect me to get in that @#$%&&*$* canoe on that @#$%&&*$* lake?"

I promise he is smarter than this will sound. And that I am just as bitchy as I will sound. In my family, we call my behavior being the bell cow, as in "She who wears the bell leads the herd—and takes no shit from other cows."

Eric answered, "Absolutely, honey. It'll be great. Here, help me get the canoe in the water. I'd take it off the car myself, but with that wind, whew, it's like a sail. Careful not to dump it over; it's reallllly cold in there. Not like that, love. Where are you going? Did I say something wrong?"

I responded by slamming the car door. Anger gave way to tears that pricked the corners of my eyes. I stewed in my thoughts. I knew I had to try to canoe. I couldn't quit before I started. We were training, and if I didn't do it, Eric wouldn't do it, and that wasn't fair of me.

I exited the car. Eric was dragging the canoe out of the water and trying to avoid looking like a red flag waving in front of me.

Super-rationally, I asked, "What are you doing?"

He said, "Well, I'm not going to make you do this."

"You're not making me. I'm scared. I hate this. I'll probably fall in and all you'll find is my frozen carcass next summer. But I'm going to do it."

My poor husband.

We paddled clockwise around the lake in the shallows, where the waves were lowest, and I fought for breath. I'm not sure if it was the constriction of all the clothing layers or actually hyperventilation, but either way, I panted like a three-hundred-pound marathoner. It would have scared off any animal life within five miles if you could have heard me over the wind. Suddenly, Eric shot me a wild-eyed look and started paddling furiously toward the center of the lake.

"You're going the wrong way!" I protested.

"I can't hear you," he shouted back.

"Turn around!"

"I can't turn around right now, I'm paddling."

"Eric Hutchins, turn the canoe back toward the shore!"

And as quickly as his mad dash for the deep had started, it stopped. He angled the canoe for the shoreline.

"What in the hell was that all about?" I asked.

"Nothing, love. I just needed to get my heart rate up."

I sensed the lie, but I couldn't prove it. My own heart raced as if I had been the one sprint-paddling. For once, though, I kept my mouth shut.

The waves grew higher. We paddled and paddled for what felt

like hours, but made little forward progress against the wicked-cold wind.

"Eric, I really want out of the canoe."

"We're halfway. Hang in there."

"No. I want out right now. I'm scared. We're going to tip over. I can't breathe."

"How about we cut across the middle of lake and shave off some distance? That will get you to the shore faster."

"I WANT TO GO THE NEAREST SHORE RIGHT NOW AND GET OUT OF THE #%$&(&^%#@% CANOE."

Now I really had to get out, because it was the second time I'd called the canoe a bad name, and I knew it would be out to get me.

Eric paddled us to the shore without another word. I'm pretty sure he thought some, but he didn't say them. I got out, almost falling over into the water and turning myself into a giant super-absorbent Tampax. He turned the canoe back over the water and continued on without me. This wasn't how I'd pictured it going down, but I knew I had better let him a) work out and b) work *me* out of his system. Looking like the Michelin man, I trudged back around the lake to the car and beat him there by only half an hour.

By the time we'd loaded the canoe onto the top of our rental car and hopped in, we were well on our way back to our happy place. Yes, I know I don't deserve him. I don't question it; I just count my blessings.

That night we dined out—did I mention we were starving to death on broccoli and whole-wheat tabbouleh?—to celebrate our marriage. Eric had arranged for flowers to be delivered to our table before we got there. The aroma was scrumptious: cow, cooked cow! Yay! And, of course, the flowers. I looked at Eric's wind-chafed, sunburned face and almost melted from the heat of adoring him. Or maybe it was from the flame of the candle, which I was huddling over to stay warm. What was wrong with the people in this state? Somebody needed to buy Montana a giant heater. We held hands and traded swipes of Chapstick.

He interrupted my moment. "I have a confession to make. And I promise you are really going to think this is funny later."

Uh oh. "Spill it, baby."

"Remember when I paddled us toward the middle of the lake as hard as I could?"

"I'm trying to block the whole experience out of my mind."

"Yeah, well, let me tell you, sweetness, it was about ten times worse for me than you. But do you remember what you said about falling in, yadda yadda, frozen carcass next summer, blah blah?"

I didn't dignify this with an answer, but he didn't need one and continued without much of a pause. "Well, you were in front of me, breathing into your paper bag or whatever, when I looked down, straight down, into the eyes and nostrils of a giant, bloated, frozen, very dead, fully intact, floating ELK CARCASS."

"You're lying."

"I am not. It was so close to the surface that if you hadn't still had those tears in your eyes, there is no way you wouldn't have seen it. You could have touched its head with your hand without even getting your wrist wet."

"No, you did NOT take me out on a lake with giant frozen dead animals floating in it." A macabre version of Alphabits cereal popped into my mind.

"Yes, I did," he said, and he hummed a few bars of Queen's "We Are the Champions."

"Oh my God. If I had seen it right then, I would have come unhinged."

"More unhinged. I know. I was terrified you would capsize us and then you would quadruple freak out in the water bumping into that thing. I had to paddle for my life."

He was right. I let him enjoy his moment; I'm glad he confessed. But I will never canoe on a tundra lake with Eric again. Even if I got my courage up, he would never invite me.

Cinderella, eat your heart out. {There's video of the tundra lake and other parts of our Montana trip on my YouTube channel, The Land of Pamelot. Sorry, there is no video of the elk.}

Click to continue reading *How to Screw Up Your Marriage.*

ACKNOWLEDGMENTS

Huge thanks to my editor Meghan Pinson, who managed to keep my ego intact without sacrificing her editorial integrity. Thanks of generous proportions to my writing group, without whose encouragement and critiques I would not be publishing this book. Lots of love to the Hotze Health and Wellness Center for giving me my life back. Big thanks and big up to "Liz, Susanne, and Clark," for all the times the triathlon and marathon training schedules didn't mesh with theirs, and for putting up with me when I was hormonal. And thanks to the power of infinity to my husband Eric for his coaching, patience, foot massages, and support.

Finally, to each and every blessed one of you who have read, reviewed, rated, and emailed/Facebooked/Tweeted/commented about my books, I appreciate you more than I can say. Stephanie, Rhonda, Liz, and Rebecca stand above the rest here. It is the readers who move mountains for me and for other authors, and I humbly ask for the honor of your honest reviews and recommendations.

BOOKS BY THE AUTHOR

Fiction from SkipJack Publishing

THE *PATRICK FLINT* SERIES OF WYOMING MYSTERIES:

Switchback (Patrick Flint #1)

Snake Oil (Patrick Flint #2)

Sawbones (Patrick Flint #3)

Scapegoat (Patrick Flint #4)

Snaggle Tooth (Patrick Flint #5)

Stag Party (Patrick Flint #6)

Sitting Duck (Patrick Flint #7)

Skin & Bones (Patrick Flint #8)

Spark (Patrick Flint 1.5): Exclusive to subscribers

THE *JENN HERRINGTON* WYOMING MYSTERIES:

BIG HORN (Jenn Herrington #1)

WALKER PRAIRIE (Jenn Herrington #2)

THE *WHAT DOESN'T KILL YOU* SUPER SERIES:

Wasted in Waco (WDKY Ensemble Prequel Novella): Exclusive to Subscribers

The Essential Guide to the What Doesn't Kill You Series

Katie Connell Caribbean Mysteries:

Saving Grace (Katie Connell #1)

HER Last CRY (Detective Delaney Pace Series Book 3)

HER Forgotten Shadow (Detective Delaney Pace Series Book 4)

Juvenile from SkipJack Publishing

Poppy Needs a Puppy (Poppy & Petey #1)

Nonfiction from SkipJack Publishing

The Clark Kent Chronicles

Hot Flashes and Half Ironmans

How to Screw Up Your Kids

How to Screw Up Your Marriage

Puppalicious and Beyond

What Kind of Loser Indie Publishes,

and How Can I Be One, Too?

Audio, e-book, large print, hardcover, and paperback versions of most titles available.

ABOUT THE AUTHOR

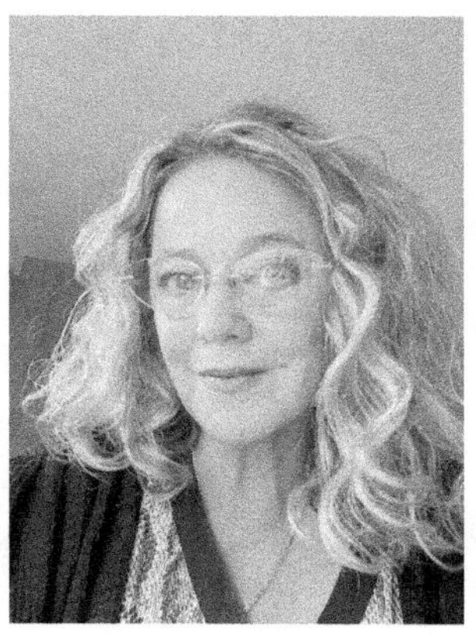

Pamela Fagan "PF" Hutchins is a *USA Today* best selling author. She writes award-winning mystery/thriller/suspense from way up in the frozen north of Snowheresville, Wyoming, where she lives with her husband in an off-the-grid cabin on the face of the Bighorn Mountains, and Mooselookville, Maine, in a rustic lake cabin. She is passionate about their large brood of kids, step kids, inherited kids, and grandkids, riding their gigantic horses, and about hiking/snow shoeing/cross country skiing/ski-joring/bike-joring/dog sledding with their Alaskan Malamutes.

If you'd like Pamela to speak to your book club, women's club, class, or writers group by streaming video or in person, shoot her an email. She's very likely to say yes.

You can connect with Pamela via her website
(http://pamelafaganhutchins.com)
or email (pamela@pamelafaganhutchins.com).

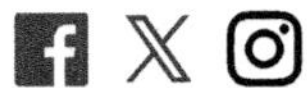

Copyright © 2012 by Pamela Fagan Hutchins

All rights reserved.

No part of this book may be reproduced in any form or by any electronic or mechanical means, including information storage and retrieval systems, without written permission from the author, except for the use of brief quotations in a book review.

To "Susanne," the female heir apparent to my hormones and genetics.
I'm sorry, honey.
If it helps any, you'll always have really great skin.

www.ingramcontent.com/pod-product-compliance
Lightning Source LLC
Chambersburg PA
CBHW070818160726
48004CB00001B/322